Pilates

for Children and Adolescents

Pilates

for Children and Adolescents

Manual of Guidelines and Curriculum

Celeste Corey-Zopich, RMT, NASM®-YES, PMA-CPT,
Chair, PMA Pilates 4 Youth Committee and Owner/Director of Pilates Staten
Island and the Center For Transformational Wellness, New York

Brett Howard, MA in Dance Education from New York University, PMA-CPT,
Director of Education for the United States Pilates Association,
Director of the Pilates Haus, New Jersey

Dawn-Marie Ickes, MPT, CNT, VMP, CST, NASM®-YES, PMA-CPT,
Adjunct DPT faculty CSUN, MSMC, Owner of Evolve Integrative Wellness,
Physical Therapy and Pilates, Orange County, CA

Contributions

Tracy Coe, PMA-CPT, Owner of Body & Mind Coe-Dynamics Inc., Manhattan Beach, CA

Editor

Tracey Mellor, BSc, RYT500, FFT, REP's L3 instructor for Pilates and yoga, Brighton, UK

Foreword by

Lolita San Miguel, Certified by Mr. Joseph Pilates in the Pilates Method of Body
Conditioning, through the Division of Vocational Rehabilitation and Training,
State University of New York, Certificate from Carola Trier, PMA-CPT

Movement photography by Al Mida, www.almida.com

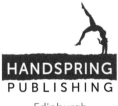

PMA
PILATES
METHOD
ALLIANCE

HANDSPRING
PUBLISHING
Edinburgh

HANDSPRING PUBLISHING LIMITED

The Old Manse, Fountainhall,
Pencaitland, East Lothian
EH34 5EY, Scotland
Tel: +44 1875 341 859
Website: www.handspringpublishing.com
First published 2014 in the United Kingdom by Handspring Publishing

ISBN 978-1-909141-12-4

British Library Cataloguing in Publication Data

A catalogue record for this book is available from the British Library

Library of Congress Cataloguing in Publication Data

A catalog record for this book is available from the Library of Congress

Notice

Neither the Publisher nor the Authors assume any responsibility for any loss, injury and/or damage to persons or property arising out of or related to any use of the information contained in this book. It is the sole responsibility of the instructor to determine appropriate and safe Pilates programming for their students.

Commissioning Editor: Sarena Wolfaard
Cover design by Gillian Murray
Illustration, Design and Page layout by Designers Collective Limited
Index by Dr Laurence Errington
Printed by Edwards Brothers Malloy, USA

Contents

SECTION ONE: TEACHING GUIDELINES

SECTION TWO: THE EXERCISE CHAPTERS

SECTION THREE: CURRICULUM

Foreword

I see in Joseph H. Pilates a formidable heir to a tradition that goes back to the Greeks and is best expressed by the Latin saying "mens sana in corpore sana," or "a sound mind in a healthy body." Physical training in ancient times was an endeavor of great prestige. Indeed, it was a national necessity to train males in intense comprehensive physical activity starting in pre-adolescence, since the life and death of human societies depended on the existence of a large population of males in superb physical condition.

We may consider ourselves "superior" in many respects to earlier societies, but in the area of physical fitness we are quite *inferior* even by the standards of only a few decades ago. According to the Centers for Disease Control and Prevention, obesity now affects 17% of all children and adolescents in the United States - triple the rate from just one generation ago. The provision of physical education in US schools is at an all time low, and in some districts is non-existent. We hear a great deal of rhetoric about a national commitment to effective physical education of our youth (especially during the "magic window" of ages 9-13). Sadly, it is only words; there is no substance. It is a national shame.

The correct education of young people about what constitutes physical fitness needs a major overhaul. Our educational system must get away from primarily sports-driven physical education for the masses. We should develop in our young people an awareness of the glorious complexity that is their body. We should teach them that like any complex machine it needs constant and proper maintenance; and that the body cannot be abused with impunity without serious consequences.

We know that early and consistent training and exposure to effective exercise will enhance posture, flexibility, strength and good health. For people so exposed, the essential routine maintenance not only becomes second nature, it becomes fun, and eventually a palpable need – even in our golden years.

In my talks around the world I often mention that the dream of Joseph Pilates was to have his Method disseminated everywhere for the good of mankind, beginning with children in schools. He knew that what he had created had great value. As his Method enlarges its reach and its influence grows, we are becoming more and more aware that this man of humble birth who died penniless was a true intuitive genius. Not only did he analyze with great precision how the human body works, most importantly he created a body of exercises to help it reach a level of excellence in flexibility and strength. In addition he created a number of apparatuses to aid in that goal and keep the human body humming at its optimum level. Many people tell me that I am a good example of the benefits of Pilates. As I write this, I am in my 80th year and my 56th year of doing Pilates, which I practice every day. I am healthy, flexible and still lead an active life with a capacity for work that many envy. One of my secrets, I must admit, is the never-ending stream of blessings I continue to receive from Spirit—the third pillar of the Body-Mind-Spirit that Pilates mentioned and which still remains to be further developed in our industry.

I am very pleased to see that, at last, a book dedicated to the teaching of the Pilates Method to children and adolescents is being published. Its aim is to provide the teacher, parent and student with the tools to live a healthy, fit life. When combined with good nutrition, the Pilates Method will change their lives for the better and is something that will remain with them for ever. Let us hope that this book with its fun attitude towards exercise will prove seminal and make decision makers take notice of the immense value and life-long impact the Pilates Method can have in the physical education of young people.

The Pilates Method for young people differs considerably from what we know as the standard Pilates teaching methodology. First of all, teachers must enjoy children: a *sine qua non*. Then they must have a keen sense of imagery, creativity and fun. This book provides exercises for the proper age levels, a varied syllabus and lots of good advice. I thank the authors and am certain this book will inspire and motivate many, including those who do not intend to engage in teaching children. Pilates is fun. Pilates *works*! Enjoy it!

Lolita San Miguel
Certified by Joseph H. Pilates through the State University of New York
Certificate from Carola Trier, PMA-CPT
Palm Beach Gardens, Florida, USA
February 2014

Preface

This book presents the fruits of more than 10 years of inspiring and rewarding work focused on bringing Pilates to young people. A guiding concern in this process has been to teach Pilates safely to children and adolescents, taking into consideration the physiological and cognitive stages of development that they undergo.

The Pilates in the Schools program and its pilot studies, which became the impetus for this book, originated at a PMA board meeting that I attended in Florida in 2002. Surrounded by visionary leaders in the Pilates world, I realized that my own background in pediatric development and rehabilitation provided a platform for demonstrating that Pilates can help children.

The first program pilot was launched in 2004 at my daughter's school and the outcome was truly astonishing. I knew what the results of Pilates had been for the many adults with whom I had worked, but had no idea how profound the effect of this work could be for children.

The response from the participants in that first pilot was heartwarming. I remember the flood of emotion that overcame me and the other three adults in the room as we stood in the cafeteria listening to the children describe how they felt different after doing Pilates. We heard numerous statements such as, "It [Pilates] is helping me with my studies because I am more relaxed, because I know that I am breathing and I am not going to tighten up," and, "It's helped me concentrate and relax more, and I'm not like, 'Oh my gosh, I have another test' and I can't really breathe. Pilates helps me relax." There were certainly many physical changes involved, but the theme of the children's unplanned, unscripted responses was one of whole-body health, decreased stress and improved ability to manage challenges.

This first pilot was the beginning of what eventually became the PMA's Pilates 4 Youth initiative, offering children and adolescents the opportunity to experience the mental, physical and emotional health benefits inherent in the Pilates Method. The absence of research in Pilates in 2002 drove the PMA to establish standards and guidelines for safe and appropriate applications of Pilates for individuals of all ages.

What follows in this book aims to provide, in words and pictures, an authoritative reference and manual for everyone working to enable children and adolescents to experience the benefits of Pilates.

Dawn-Marie Ickes, Orange County, CA. February 2014

Acknowledgments

I would like to express my deep appreciation for the work of the authors and contributors to this book, which represents ten years of investigation, exploration and effort in teaching Pilates safely and effectively to young people. There are also many others, not named here, who undertook pilot investigations and participated in committee work over the past decade in the name of making Joseph Pilates' goal of teaching his exercise method to young people a reality. I extend my sincere thanks to all who contributed.

Specifically, I would like to thank ...

PMA co-founder Kevin Bowen, who believes strongly in the importance of promoting Pilates for children. Mr. Bowen established the PMA's original Pilates in the Schools program and committee in 2003, and lobbied legislators in Washington D.C. to promote the many benefits of the Pilates Method for both adults and young people.

Dawn-Marie Ickes, for directing the PMA's Pilates in the Schools program from 2003 to 2009, and for correlating proven health and wellness practices with the application of Pilates for children and adolescents. The Pilates in the Schools program provided the framework for a series of pilot studies of the efficacy of Pilates for children, focusing on the 9 to 13 age group.

Celeste Corey-Zopich, for her leadership, beginning in 2009, of the PMA's Pilates 4 Youth initiative and committee, focusing on the creation of effective guidelines for teaching Pilates to young people ages 5 to 18; and for providing the impetus and momentum that resulted in the creation of this book.

Brett Howard, for contributing his expertise in the field of education and the teaching of Pilates to young people.

Kyria Sabin, for coordinating the production of photographs of young people for this book.

Jeremy Wallace, for the creation and production of the Pilates in The Schools: Program Pilot DVD, in 2005.

Sherri Betz and Shelly Power, for their invaluable advice and encouragement.

Elizabeth Anderson, Executive Director, Pilates Method Alliance, 2014

Dedication

This book is dedicated to the late Joseph H. Pilates, whose clear and far-reaching vision for health and well-being sustains us today. May this book contribute to the achievement of his goal to "First educate the child!"

Pilates Method Alliance

The Pilates Method Alliance (PMA) is the international, not-for-profit, professional association and certifying agency dedicated to the teachings of Joseph H. and Clara Pilates. The PMA is a 501(c)(3) organization incorporated in the State of Florida, USA.

www.pilatesmethodalliance.org and info@pilatesmethodalliance.org

Introduction

The Pilates 4 Youth initiative was created to address young people's fitness, health and overall well-being. As an outgrowth of the initiative, this manual and curriculum have been designed as a resource for Pilates teachers, educators, families, and community leaders interested in using the Pilates Method for the improved physical, mental, emotional, and social health of young people. The manual discusses a spectrum of relevant topics, such as child and adolescent growth and development, factors supporting students' well-being and positive outcomes, safe practices and ethics, teaching considerations, and age-appropriate Pilates exercise practice. Additionally, there are two sample curriculums that can be adapted and used in conjunction with the manual by those interested in working in a formal school setting.

Why Pilates for Young People?

Joseph Hubertus Pilates, founder of the Pilates Method, believed that we must "First educate the child." His method, originally termed "Contrology," promotes the principles of an integrated body and mind, and recommends beginning the practice at a young age.

> "In childhood, habits are easily formed – good and bad. Why not then concentrate on the formation of only good habits and thus avoid the necessity later on in life of attempting to correct bad habits and substituting for them good habits."
>
> (Pilates, 1934)

Factors affecting young people's health today include not only physical inactivity, due to increased sedentary behavior in a world of smart phones, video gaming, computer activities, and TV watching (CDC, 2003–2006), but also, more alarmingly, decreased emphasis on, and varying mandates for, physical education programming in schools. In addition, we see unhealthy dietary behavior in general, such as large portions of food with little nutritional value, and a high percentage of school environments that allow for the purchase of unhealthy foods and beverages (sweets, high-fat snacks, soft drinks, and sports drinks). These factors contribute to placing our youth at risk for becoming the first generation to have shorter lifespans than their parents.

In the United States, the negative trend in young people's health is so prevalent that the current presidential administration has developed the *Let's Move!* initiative as a platform for tackling this issue. The US Centers for Disease Control (CDC), the American Heart Association, and the National Association for Sports and Physical Education all recommend daily physical education from kindergarten through the end of high school. At the present time, daily physical education is not part of many school curriculums in the US, and this fact is coupled with an overall decline in general physical activity.

If "Physical fitness is the first requisite of happiness," as Joseph Pilates believed, and if young people's wellness is suffering due to lack of physical activity, interventions to correct this should be considered a mandate. The beauty of the Pilates Method and the offerings of this manual are that they can be practiced anywhere – in a school, home, youth center, or studio. Physical activity such as Pilates fosters neurological development and a deepening integration of the mind and body. Our brain structure and development are intimately connected to the movement mechanisms within our body (Hannaford, 2005).

It has been proven that physical activity during childhood and adolescence can exert both direct and indirect positive effects on adult health (Dumith, 2012). There is strong evidence of positive physical markers in young people that are related to regular physical activity. These are shown in body composition, cardiorespiratory and muscular fitness, bone health, and metabolic health. Above and beyond the physical markers, cognitive data shows that physical activity in young people is consistently related to higher levels of self-esteem, and lower levels of anxiety and stress. It is also relevant to note that young people who participate in a variety of physical activities develop better cognitive and motor skills and increase their self-confidence and self-efficacy.

Bringing Pilates to Young People

It is crucial for all children to be exposed to physical activities that offer opportunities for successful movement experiences. Research suggests that boys generally have a higher probability of increased physical activity from middle school onward, whereas girls tend to decrease or stop their involvement in physical activity at this time. These changes in exercise patterns happen during the transition from elementary to middle school (Liu et al., 2012). It is this stage, from the ages of 9 to 13, which we define as the "Magic Window". The Magic Window concept was conceived by Dawn-Marie Ickes for the PMA's Pilates in the Schools program pilots, and denotes the optimal age range for introducing an exercise modality such as Pilates. The Magic Window occurs just before the skeletal and muscular growth spurts that come with puberty, when young people in this age group are at the peak of neurological development. Learning effective and functional movement during these years of neurological development can foster an improvement in "perception" of physical abilities (Marcus, 2003). When we prioritize the mind-body connection experiences of young people, we are preparing them for success later in life.

Pilates stated that, "Civilization impairs physical fitness." He created his method to "develop the body uniformly, correct wrong postures, restore physical vitality, invigorate the mind and elevate the spirit."

With regard to young people's health, Pilates exercises can:

1. Override the body's physiological response to stress.
2. Initiate the relaxation response and invigorate the nervous system by means of concentrated and focused breathing.
3. Integrate all the body's systems to bring students into an energized, alert state.
4. Organize whole brain function for optimal learning.
5. Raise levels of all chemical "messengers" known to balance behavior and inhibit hunger.
6. Unify the cognitive and motor regions of the brain critical to strengthening our attention and coordination, by the introduction of cross-lateral movements.
7. Create a fun, harmonious, and safe way of learning and developing group dynamics and social skills.
8. Reduce stress, increase mind and body fitness, and develop key elements of lifetime health such as:
   a. Self-awareness.
   b. Self-care and self-management.

Pilates is a unique practice that focuses on foundational and functional movement skills, which challenges and stimulates the student while integrating the body and mind through a series of specific exercises. With this in mind, Pilates can be taught in a manner that is fun for young people, and it readily complements traditional exercise regimens taught in schools.

The Mat exercises presented in this manual can be practiced in 10-minute, 20-minute, 30-minute, or 45-minute modules, or any variation thereof. They represent a small percentage of the complete method, but offer the most accessible format for working with young people. Utilizing Pilates Mat exercises, or floor-based exercise, young participants in a variety of teaching environments can experience this amazing life enhancing exercise method. It is a practice for everyone, which can be done almost anywhere.

This manual offers chapters on specific age groups, in order to target their particular physical and learning capacities, as well as to optimize their growth and development needs. Additionally, the manual offers modifications and progressions for safe execution at any level. Pilates approaches wellness by looking at both the body and mind – the whole person. Young people engaging in Pilates Mat work learn physical skills while incorporating body awareness through disciplined focus, concentration, coordination, healthy breathing, mindful and controlled movement. Pilates promotes the connection between building strength and flexibility on the one hand, and developing conscious awareness of the body on the other.

Ultimately, the practice of Pilates fosters excellence in mental fitness, emotional intelligence, physical well-being, and social competence.

The PMA's Pilates in the Schools program pilots, initiated by the pioneering work of Dawn Marie-Ickes and carried out by independent teachers throughout the US, ran for six years, and confirmed that students respond positively to the opportunity to learn about their bodies and the mind-body connection. These pilots revealed that, in addition to the measured benefits of improved balance, core strength, and flexibility, students identified an improved ability to manage anxiety and stress, and gained the ability to self-regulate. Benefits of this sort carry over into the lives of young people, and impact their participation in school, in sports, in activities at home, and in society. Appendix 1 at the end of this manual provides more detail on the pilots and their outcomes.

Manual Content

This manual discusses important considerations for teaching Pilates to young people, particularly with regard to physiological and psychosocial development. It is vital to remember that children are not miniature adults (AAP, 2001), and Pilates programming must reflect this fact on all levels. The manual contains a full exploration of physiology and development for young people, from early childhood (ages 2-6) through adolescence (ages 12-18). Chapter 1 presents information on physiological development, comprising bone and growth plate development, thermoregulation, breathing, posture, and flexibility. The chapter also features a discussion of growth plate injuries and bone health. It then delineates additional developmental considerations for each age group.

Chapter 2 discusses the factors surrounding young people's well-being, and considerations for positive outcomes. This chapter emphasizes that in order to work effectively with young people, it is necessary to know more than physiology. There are also cognitive factors that influence young people and their capacity for positive outcomes and achievement. This chapter highlights the concepts of "self-esteem", "self-efficacy", and "self-perception," and presents teaching strategies and principles of achievement to inform the

Pilates teachers approach to working with young people.

Chapter 3 discusses the age group of 9 to 13 (the Magic Window) as the optimal time to introduce Pilates to young people and to offer an experience that can foster healthy habits for life.

Chapter 4 is devoted to the teacher. This chapter is about pedagogy – the art and science of teaching – and highlights important considerations for successful teaching practice when working with young people.

Chapter 5 concerns general procedures within the teaching environment, safety, and professionalism, and outlines necessary considerations for working with young people in any setting. Included here is information on liability insurance, administrative forms, and first aid, as well as professional scope of practice and ethics, and the position of the Pilates teacher as a role model.

Chapter 6 through 9 comprise the formal exercise chapters.

There is a chapter for Pre-Pilates exercises, which offers fundamental movements that introduce breathing awareness, pelvic awareness, cervical awareness, rib cage awareness, shoulder girdle awareness, spinal mobility and core stability.

There are dedicated chapters with exercise programming for:

- 5–8 year-olds, (ideally taught by credentialed early childhood education practitioners)
- 9–13-year-olds (middle childhood and early adolescence)
- 12–18-year-olds (adolescence)

Chapter 10 is intended for Pilates teachers who are interested in teaching within a school environment. This section addresses the question of how to make an effective Pilates curriculum presentation to a school administrator, and comprises topics such as what a curriculum is, why it is needed, how it should be presented for the best chance of acceptance, and its essential components. Two sample curriculums have been included as examples of how a curriculum presentation can be made. We hope that this material will equip Pilates teachers wishing to work at their local schools with an understanding of how to present a Pilates curriculum to school administrators for the best chance of success.

The PMA has developed this manual as a resource to support Pilates teachers who have a particular interest in working with children and adolescents. Our young people have much to gain by learning an exercise method that can aid in "the attainment and maintenance of a uniformly developed body with a sound mind fully capable of naturally, easily, and satisfactorily performing our many and varied daily tasks with spontaneous zest and pleasure" (Pilates, 1945).

Pilates is for everyone, and it is our hope to bring Joseph Pilates' dream to fruition and inspire the youth of today to be the Pilates practitioners of tomorrow.

References

American Academy of Pediatrics (AAP)., 2001. Strength training by children and adolescents. *Pediatrics*,107(6):1470–1472. [Online] Available at: http://pediatrics.aappublications.org/content/121/4/835

CDC National Center for Health Statistics, Health E-Stat. NHANES. 2003-2006. Data on the prevalence of overweight among children and adolescents: United States. [Online] Available at: http://www.cdc.gov/nchs/products/pubs/pubd/hestats/overweight/overwght_child_03.htm.

Dumith, S. C. et al., 2012. A longitudinal evaluation of physical activity in Brazilian adolescents: tracking, change and predictors. *Pediatric Exercise Science*, 24(1):58–71

Hannaford, Carla., 2005. *Smart moves: why learning is not all in your head.* Salt Lake City, UT: Great River Books

Liu, W. et al., 2012. Tracking of health-related physical fitness for middle school boys and girls. *Pediatric Exercise Science*, 24(4):549–562

Marcus, B. H., Forsyth, L. H., 2003. *Motivating people to be physically active.* Champaign, IL: Human Kinetics

Pilates, J. H. , 1934. *Your health.* Reprinted in: A Pilates' primer: The millennium edition. Incline Village, NV: Presentation Dynamics Inc.

Pilates, J. H., 2005. *Pilates' Return to Life Through Contrology.* Miami, FL: Pilates Method Alliance; Originally published in 1945

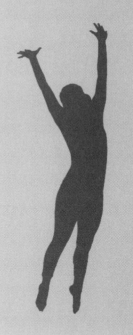

Section One
Teaching Guidelines

Chapter 1
Physiology and Development

The exponential growth of the Pilates Method in the past 15 years has created the opportunity for individuals of all ages, shapes, and sizes to experience this approach to healthy, integrative, and whole body movement. The rise in interest for programming specifically geared towards young people has prompted the creation of instructional guidelines for Pilates teachers, based on globally accepted developmental norms for children and adolescents.

Working with children and adolescents is wonderfully challenging for Pilates teachers, as we are compelled to realize that we are *not* working with a smaller version of an adult. As they grow and mature, young people undergo a series of changes-- neurologically, skeletally, muscularly, hormonally, and emotionally. Teaching young people, who are in the process of undergoing these changes, is dramatically different from teaching adults who are fully mature. It is difficult to predict the pace of these changes with any accuracy, because there is considerable variance within each of the body's systems, as well as within each individual child. Many changes are not readily observable simply by looking at the child or adolescent.

This chapter provides an overview of the physiological and developmental changes that young people experience on their way to becoming adults. Recognizing these changes will provide a solid foundation for the development of Pilates programming for young people that is safe, adaptable, progressive, effective, and fun!

Common Physiological Considerations

Bone and growth plate development

The *growth plate*, also known as the epiphyseal plate, is a plate of *cartilage* that allows growth to occur. In long bones, the growth plates lie between the epiphysis (end of the bone), and the diaphysis (shaft of the bone) (Patton, 2009). They also exist within the vertebrae. Growth plates are vulnerable to injury (fractures) during childhood and adolescence. They are also found in other bones in the body, but the long bones and vertebrae are the sites that concern us most as teachers of Pilates working with young people.

Understanding bone and growth plate development is the most important consideration when teaching Pilates to young people. In order for teachers to create safe and appropriate exercise programs, they must understand both how the bone structure of an adult is different from that of a child and the effects of excessive stress on the growth plates.

From a structural perspective, a child's bones are more porous and flexible than an adult's, resulting in increased susceptibility to fractures (McCance, 2010). Growth plates in particular are at increased risk due to the sensitive nature of this area of the bone. Injuries that would only cause joint sprains in adults can cause more serious injury in young people. The bones of a child grow continuously, sometimes very slowly and at other times in spurts, the latter particularly during puberty. During growth spurts, the risk of overtraining is at its peak. Bones can grow faster than the muscles and connective tissue are able to adapt, and, as a result, the tendons may become inflamed at their insertions.

The incidence of sports injuries in young people has increased exponentially since 2002 and continues to show a rising trend as a result of training practices that do not account for the challenges that growth spurts present (Hoang, 2012). Special caution when applying the principles of Pilates to the musculoskeletal imbalances seen in young people is warranted to ensure that programs are safe and effective.

Thermoregulation

Thermoregulation is the regulation of body temperature.

A child's body regulates its temperature differently from an adult's, both during exercise and at rest (Malina, 2004; Rowland, 2005). For example, as total body water and blood volume are lower in children than in adults because of their smaller size, there is a smaller reserve volume when fluid loss occurs. The child's greater metabolic rate means that children heat up more rapidly than adults. Also, due to a child's higher surface area to mass ratio, their core temperature rises more quickly than an adult's does. In hot weather, children may have difficulty dissipating heat, and they may lose heat too quickly in cold environments where skin is exposed, such as in swimming (NASM, 2012). As such, it is important for the teacher to observe and respond appropriately to the child's reaction to exercise, including its effects on their complexion (increased redness or paleness), breathing rates and perspiration. The teacher must also take into account the temperature both inside and outside of the teaching facility, as dramatic changes in temperature or extremes of temperature can impact the students and their response to exercise. Appropriate clothing is essential, based on the temperature of the classroom, as are sufficient water breaks during the class.

Breathing

Breathing (or ventilation) involves the mechanical movement of gases into and out of the lungs. Respiration is the process of gas exchange within the lungs (Hillegass, 2011).

The lungs are not fully developed until the end of puberty in males and at menarche in females. Lung development impacts minute ventilation (volume of gas inhaled or exhaled from a person's lungs per minute) and tidal volume (volume of air displaced between normal inspiration and expiration when extra effort is not applied) (Nève, 2002). The number of breaths per minute is greater for children and adolescents than for adults, because the lungs of young people are still developing and they have a greater requirement for oxygenation (Nève, 2002; NASM, 2012).

Teachers must recognize that breathing patterns for young people may be markedly different from their own, especially during movement. For example, it is to be expected that the number of breaths per minute will increase during the initial phase of physical challenge more in children and adolescents than adults.

Teaching Pilates to young people involves encouraging students to learn about their breathing patterns, to become aware of the coordination of breath with movement, and to appreciate how breathing with awareness can promote respiratory efficiency and support the demands of their growing bodies.

When young people learn to intentionally coordinate breathing with movement, this ability can positively impact many of their future endeavors, from sports and recreational activities to academic and competitive cognitive challenges.

Considerations for Teaching

Posture

Posture is an essential aspect of whole-body health. It is often looked at from a static perspective, such as assessing how a person stands, and is commonly evaluated from this static viewpoint.

A more accurate viewpoint is that posture is both static and dynamic. It can include the natural way one stands, moves into and out of positions, or assumes a pose, and it is present in all movement.

Posture may be assessed as 'optimal' or 'imbalanced'. Optimal posture is generally the result of efficient use of the body's musculoskeletal structure, providing the internal tissues, organs, and systems the space they require for good, balanced function. Optimal posture promotes an integrated use of the entire body. Imbalanced posture can lead to musculoskeletal inefficiency, which may cause biomechanical problems, spinal irregularities and pain.

Evaluating posture in young people – both children and adolescents – is very different from evaluating posture in an adult. While children are still growing, their dynamic and static postures are continuously changing.

The list below highlights postural norms for young people as defined by Florence Kendall. By understanding postural norms, the teacher can recognize deviations and focus on specific postural corrections (Kendall, 2005).

Postural norms for young people:

The feet
- It is common for the arch of the foot to appear flat until the age of 6 or 7, when arch formation becomes more visible.

The knees
- Both hyperextension and knock-knees are common in children.
- Hyperextension should resolve as the ligaments tighten, but often persists as a postural habit.
- Knock-knees usually diminish by the age of 6 or 7.

The neck and trunk
- Young children have a significant imbalance between the strength of the anterior and posterior muscles of the neck and trunk, which begins in infancy and diminishes over time. For example, the head position for The Hundred is more challenging for a child than for an adult.
- It is not uncommon for a small child to have a protruding abdomen, which decreases between the ages of 10 and 12 as the muscles become more developed.
- Children exhibit many variations in standing posture. Early school-age children commonly have a postural deviation where their shoulder blades protrude. Beginning around age 9, increased lumbar lordosis, or curve, is noticeable. These deviations should become less pronounced as the child grows.
- The normal range of motion for both lumbar flexion and extension decreases from childhood onward.

Growth spurts
- During a growth spurt, posture may be imbalanced for a period of time for the young person, because bones, tendons and muscles tend to grow at different rates.

Adolescence

- Cases of hypermobility (excessive joint mobility) or hypomobility (restricted joint mobility) may continue into adolescence. Working with each student individually to achieve balanced flexibility in each given exercise will assist in correcting any imbalances such conditions may create.

Anticipating some of the common postural issues a young person may encounter is helpful for developing appropriate programming for all age groups.

Flexibility

Flexibility is defined as the range of motion around a joint (Magee, 2011). Balanced flexibility, or flexibility that is balanced on both sides of a joint, is a key contributor to the proper development of joint and muscle function.

Balanced flexibility serves an important function for the neuromuscular development of a growing body and is a necessary component of any physical endeavor a young person may participate in.

It is normal for a young person's flexibility to vary as they grow and mature. For example, from ages 1 to 10, most children are able sit with their legs extended and touch their fingertips to their toes. It is perfectly normal for young people between the ages of 11 and 14 to lose some of their flexibility due to growth spurts and other physiological changes associated with puberty, and to lose their ability to touch their toes during this phase. Overstretching during puberty, when there is an observable reduction in range of motion, can lead to muscle and tendon injuries in young people and unstable joints later in life. Therefore, stretching practices that aggressively target increasing flexibility are not recommended during growth spurts (Anderson and Twist, 2005). Balanced flexibility coupled with balanced muscular development are critical components of healthy joint function and mechanics, which inherently influence posture.

Ideally, the pre-pubescent child should learn slow and controlled movements through full available ranges of motion. Although data on optimal stretching practices for young people is limited, the goal of programming for children going through puberty is to create balanced flexibility.

Growth Plate Injuries

Growth plate injuries account for approximately 30% of bone related injuries in children and adolescents (Caine, et al., 2006). Injury to the growth plate may lead to compromised bone development.

Growth plate injuries are typically caused by overuse or trauma during the growing phase of the bone. Overuse is the result of excessive training without adequate rest, and most commonly occurs in activities such as football, long distance running, gymnastics and baseball. In the process of growth, muscles and connective tissue adapt and lengthen at a slower rate than long bones do, which puts the growth plate and cartilage at risk, and the growth plate is the structure most vulnerable to injury. The most common places for growth plate injuries include the proximal humerus, distal radius, lumbar spine, tibia, and fibula.

These physiological considerations support our recommendation that programming for 8 to 13-year-olds should avoid excessive stretching.

The following areas of the body require specific consideration when teaching Pilates to young people:

The Spine

Growth plates are located near both surfaces of the vertebral body.

Growth plates appear between the ages of 8 and 12 and begin to fuse into bone following puberty. The most vulnerable time for injury is when fusion starts to take place, between the ages of 14 and 16.

Programming should avoid inversion exercises like The Jack-Knife and The Roll-Over during the middle teen years, as these exercises load the spine during a time when growth plate fusion is still occurring.

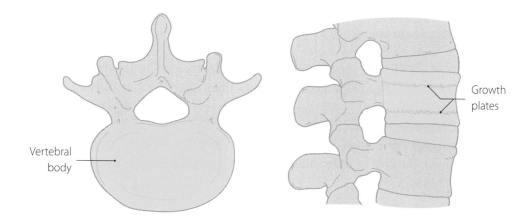

Figure 1.1 Growth plates are located near the upper and lower surfaces of the vertebral body

The complete fusion of the spinal growth plates is not complete until between 20 and 25 years of age (Marchiori, 2005). Avoiding inversion exercises until this time is the safest recommendation until further studies are performed.

The Pelvis

Damage to the pelvic region often occurs following a quick or abrupt muscle contraction, such as those experienced when changing direction in football or basketball. If damage to this area has been reported, clearance from the child's pediatrician should be obtained prior to their participation in physical activities.

The Knee

The end, or insertion, of the patellar tendon is a common place for growth plate injuries, particularly for students who participate in running-based activities. Both Sinding Larsen–Johansson and Osgood–Schlatter injuries are considered "avulsion injuries". Avulsion injuries occur when the tendon or ligament pulls away from the bone, and can arise during or after a period of growth in which the bones grow faster than the tendon. If a diagnosis of avulsion injury is reported, clearance from the child's pediatrician should be obtained prior to their participation in physical activities.

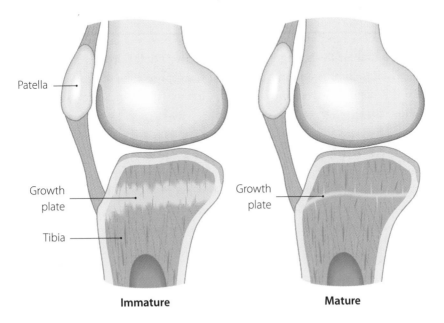

Figure 1.2 Growth plate injuries and traumas are not uncommon in young people

The Ankle

The Achilles tendon attaches to the calcaneus, or heel bone, and is frequently impacted by growth spurts. Heel pain and calf tightness are common complaints if inflammation occurs in this region during growth. In this case, caution when teaching exercises which stretch the calf muscles or the bottom of the foot is recommended.

Bone Health

Good bone density is a component of bone strength and health, and is promoted by weight-bearing physical activity. Bone is most responsive to the benefits of weight-bearing physical activity such as running or jumping prior to puberty. Bone and its mineral content develop at an increased rate during puberty, compared to early childhood.

In females, the most critical period of increase in bone density occurs prior to menarche (Mirtz et al., 2011). Stress fractures are common in females with delayed menarche or amenorrhea due to hormonal imbalances. Encouraging safe and appropriate exercise during a growth spurt and as females approach menarche optimizes bone density.

Developmental Changes by Age Group

Understanding the developmental changes in early childhood, middle childhood and adolescence is essential for designing a safe and effective Pilates program. In the headings below, we have used Solomon's definitions of the stages and ages of development. Please note that there is a degree of overlap in the way that age groupings are discussed in this manual (Solomon, 2011).

Early Childhood (Ages 2–6)

Few Pilates exercises are appropriate for early childhood; however, appropriate selections for children ages 5 to 8 are included in Chapter 7 of this manual. Teaching this group requires playful creativity, and cannot be based on learning by rote. Creative, natural variations of movement can be combined with Pilates principles to create classes for this age group.

Middle Childhood (Ages 7–11)
and Early Adolescence (Ages 12–14)

Following the rapid growth of early childhood, the rate of physical development slows down through middle childhood and early adolescence. As physical development slows, young people have the opportunity to refine many of their gross motor skills. The periods of middle childhood and early adolescence represent the optimal developmental stage for the introduction of mind-body movement education such as Pilates.

The term "Magic Window", which appears throughout this manual, was coined to identify children between the ages of 9 and 13. The "Magic Window" is a period during which the nervous system is in a highly adaptable state prior to puberty. At this time, teachers can introduce complex movements that utilize cross-lateral strategies and advanced neuromuscular coordination. When working with the "Magic Window" group, teaching the exercises in progressive stages allows the teacher to build increasingly sophisticated levels of coordination.

Adolescence (Ages 12–18)

Adolescence is the transition period between childhood and adulthood. Although this manual will discuss adolescence as reflecting the ages of 12 to 18, it should be remembered that the onset of puberty may begin before the age of 12 for some children.

Puberty generally lasts from 12 to 18 months. During this period, growth spurts occur and significant hormonal changes impact the skeletal, neurological and muscular systems. Hormonal changes can create mood shifts, body changes and increased self-consciousness. At this time there is also a general decrease in flexibility and overall range of motion. These changes produce uneven growth patterns of muscles, bones, tendons, and ligaments, which ultimately affect overall posture. This process may leave a child in an imbalanced state regarding movement, control, balance and coordination. Additionally, these changes can influence self-perception. Adolescents may experience difficulty with new activities and/or previously mastered activities, as their bodies are transforming. It is very common for an adolescent to have a shift in their kinesthetic awareness (perception of position and movement of body parts) during this time.

Appropriate exercise programming and feedback during the learning process is one means whereby young people can experience a sense of success during this 12- to 18-month period. Lesson planning which highlights the re-patterning of already familiar movements with a strong focus on body posture, awareness and muscle balance provides encouragement and support during this time (Thompson, 2003).

Pilates is especially relevant during puberty, as it highlights coordination and balance with control. It also offers flexibility that is functional and unforced. Young people going through puberty can safely practice many Pilates exercises; however, they are not physiologically developed enough to practice the full adult repertoire without risk.

Although adolescents are physiologically more developed than children in early and middle childhood, they have not yet reached full skeletal maturity. Adolescents are at risk for overtraining, due to continued muscular development and skeletal growth. Young people in this group are particularly prone to developing injuries through sports activities where training techniques do not integrate strength, flexibility, endurance, balance and coordination skills. Exercise in general can be functionally based for this group, but there is great value in incorporating movement experiences that focus on the mind–body connection. Proper programming can create efficient athleticism through whole body coordination. The repertoire of Pilates exercises for adolescents is much larger than for children in early and middle childhood, but still does not include the complete adult repertoire.

Conclusion

Pilates programs based on sound principles of childhood physiology and development can create an opportunity for young people to learn about how their minds and bodies function as an integrated whole.

The physical differences between young people and adults are fairly straightforward and easy to apply to Pilates programming. Once a solid understanding of these differences is attained, the next step is to become attuned to the mental and emotional needs of children and adolescents. Chapter 2 will explore young people's well-being and the various factors which affect this aspect of their health.

References

Anderson, G., Twist, P., 2005. Trainability of Children. *IDEA Fitness Journal.* March

Caine, D., DiFiori, J., and Maffulli, N., 2006. Physeal injuries in children's and youth sports: reasons for concern? *British Journal of Sports Medicine.* 40(9): 749-760

Hillegass, E., 2011. *Essentials of Cardiopulmonary Physical Therapy*, 3rd ed. Philadelphia: W.B. Saunders Company

Hoang QB, Mortazavi M., 2012. Pediatric overuse injuries in sports. *Advances in Pediatrics.* 2012; 59(1): 359-83

Kendall, F. P. et al., 2005. *Muscles: testing and function with posture and pain.* 5th ed. Philadelphia: Lippincott, Williams and Wilkins

Magee, D.J., 2011. *Athletic and Sport Issues in Musculoskeletal Rehabilitation.* Philadelphia: W.B.Saunders Company

Malina, R. M. et al., 2004. *Growth, maturation, and physical activity.* Champaign, IL: Human Kinetics

Marchiori, D., 2005. *Clinical imaging.* 2nd ed. St Louis, MO: Mosby

McCance, K. L., 2010. *Pathophysiology: the biologic basis for disease in adults and children.* 6th ed. St. Louis, MO: Mosby

Mirtz, T. A. et al., 2011.The effects of physical activity on the epiphyseal growth plates: A review of the literature on normal physiology and clinical implications. *Journal of Clinical Medicine Research*; 3(1):1–7

National Academy of Sports Medicine, 2012. *Youth Exercise Specialist Manual.* Assessment, Technologies Institute, LLC

Nève, V., Girard, F., Flahault, A., Boulé, M., 2002. Lung and thorax development during adolescence: relationship with pubertal status. *European Respiratory Journal*, 20: 1292–1298

Patton, Kevin T., 2009. *Anatomy & Physiology* (with Media), 7th ed. St. Louis, MO: Mosby

Rowland, T. W., 2005. *Children's exercise physiology.* Champaign, IL: Human Kinetics

Thompson, Jim., 2003. *The Double Goal Coach: Positive Coaching Tools for Honoring The Game and Developing Winners in Sports and Life.* Harper Collins

Solomon, J., O'Brien, J., 2011. *Pediatric Skills for Occupational Therapy Assistants*, 3rd ed. St. Louis, MO: Mosby

Chapter 2
Pilates and Young People's Well-Being

The differences between adults' bodies and children's bodies do not end with physiology. There are also psychosocial and emotional considerations when teaching Pilates to children.

As a fundamental principle, mental and emotional well-being are essential to overall health. Therefore, in teaching Pilates to young people, consideration for their well-being guides effective practice. Although this topic isn't addressed in Pilates manuals aimed at adults, it is an important element of teaching Pilates to children and adolescents.

Positive experiences in childhood have been shown to foster early emotional well-being. Such experiences can directly impact overall health and well-being and influence how individuals realize their full potential, cope with the stresses of life, work productively, and make meaningful contributions to their communities (National Prevention, Health Promotion and Public Health Council, 2010). Teaching Pilates to children provides an opportunity for early positive movement experiences, and has been shown to assist children with concentration, stress management, and confidence in their physicality (Ickes, 2006).

As a related point, in its definition of "quality of life", The National Academy of Sports Medicine equates quality of life with well-being: "Quality of life consists of social, emotional, psychological, and physical well-being" (NASM, 2012). Pilates teachers interested in working with children and adolescents should consider not only that they have an influence on their students' well-being, but that young people come into the teaching environment with unique backgrounds that influence their ability to interact and participate in classes.

With all of the above in mind, it is helpful to explore the different factors surrounding well-being for children and adolescents within the teaching environment, together with strategies for encouraging achievement and success.

The following are important areas for consideration.

Cognitive Factors

Self-perception, or how individuals perceive themselves, has two important components: "self-efficacy" and "self-esteem" (NASM, 2012). A young person's self-perception strongly influences achievement outcomes, as well as how he or she manages expectations and copes with challenges.

"Self-efficacy" is the measure of a person's ability to complete tasks and reach goals. It is influenced by comfort levels, expectations, and personal experience. A young person trying a new fitness activity may not have a high sense of self-efficacy. He or she may be unwilling to try or may give up easily, especially if they perceive that there are challenges or barriers they cannot overcome. Similarly, if a child believes him- or herself to be fit and capable, they may look at the new activity with a sense of confidence and willingness. "Self-esteem" is defined as a realistic respect for oneself or a favorable impression of oneself. Self-esteem equates with self-respect and feelings of worth. In the realm of fitness and health, "body competence" and "body image" are both part of self-esteem.

Body competence refers to a person's competence when participating in a physical activity. Body image is a subjective picture of one's own physical appearance, and is influenced by various factors, including a person's self-assessment, social standards of physical attractiveness, and the perceptions of others. A distorted or negative body image can lead to unhealthy behaviors and disorders, such as anorexia nervosa and body dysmorphic disorder. Self-perception, self-efficacy and self-esteem all have a direct impact on quality of life.

When beginning Pilates training with young people, highlighting both short-term and long-term expectations for all participants can help achieve a positive outcome.

For example, teachers can talk with students about the many benefits of being physically active, and the negative consequences of inactivity or a sedentary lifestyle. They can amplify students' understanding of the activities being offered to them, and the results of participating. If a child is sports-minded, the teacher can explain how Pilates will help them in their respective sport.

Teachers can influence how a student responds to class activities as well as to challenges they may face in encountering something new, such as a new exercise. Input from the teacher can:

- help the child deal with their physiological changes, or with social or peer pressure.
- build confidence and provide reassurance by demonstrating ways to modify an exercise to overcome a challenge.
- encourage an individual in the group to help motivate others and have the young people take turns demonstrating an exercise. After doing so, they can discuss how it felt, what was easy, what was hard, and, if a correction was given, how the correction helped. This approach positively motivates others to improve their form and technique, and simultaneously strengthens their self-awareness skills.

Teaching Strategies

The following are some general teaching methods suggested in *Physical Activity Interventions in Children and Adolescents* by Ward, Saunders, and Pate (2007), which we have found useful and have modified for teaching Pilates to children and adolescents. These methods are ways of providing the student with a successful experience that will enhance self-efficacy and self-esteem.

Modeling: Providing a demonstration of an exercise that an individual attempts to imitate.

Goal-setting: Establishing *specific, measurable, achievable, realistic and time-targeted* goals (SMART goals). It is important for young people that goals be realistic, based on their skill levels, and re-assessed as their skills improve.

Guided practice: An activity that provides students the opportunity to grasp and develop concepts or skills, and requires teachers to monitor student progress and offer feedback.

Imagery: The use of descriptive and vivid language. Imagery is a valuable tool and is useful in teaching Pilates to young people.

Reinforcement: Anything that strengthens or increases the likelihood of a specific behavior.

Principles of Achievement

The National Academy of Sports Medicine provides us with specific characteristics of individuals who are high achievers and are successful in making lifestyle changes.

Vision: Having a clear sense of what you want

High achievers tend to have a very clear vision and understanding of what they want to achieve and why. Research has shown that these individuals also demonstrate better psychological and physical health than those without clear goals. (Kraus, 2002; Emmons, 1988) As teachers, it is important for us to recognize that, for the most part, "vision" for children and adolescents will have a relatively short-term focus.

Strategy: Determining action steps for the achievement of goals

The best strategies for young people are those that align with their priorities and values. Strategies with this focus will maximize performance and confidence. In other words, a goal must be something the young person *wants to* achieve, as opposed to something they *have to* achieve.

Self-belief: Belief in oneself and one's ability to succeed

Belief in oneself gives rise to motivation and achievement. Encouraging students to take small steps and to recognize small achievements shows them that their goals are attainable. Success from previous experiences fosters an internal sense that achievement is possible.

Persistence: The ability to 'stay the course' in any activity

Encouraging persistence when teaching new movement skills helps the student to achieve their goals and experience their accomplishment. Providing support, compliments and appropriate rewards encourage young people to keep motivated and moving toward their goals.

Self-monitoring: Assessing one's own progress toward goals and making relevant adjustments

Assisting students in identifying progress toward or away from their goals is helpful in giving them a sense of control, competence and confidence in their endeavors.

An open and non-judgmental learning environment, together with self-monitoring, promotes achievement.

Conclusion

The well-being of students is an essential element of a positive learning experience for young people. The teacher's interaction with students must be such as to support both their self-efficacy and self-esteem, and to allow them to experience the satisfaction of accomplishing specific goals.

An understanding of teaching strategies and an awareness of the principles of achievement will guide the development of programs that foster positive outcomes for young people.

The following chapter discusses the stages of childhood and adolescent development as they pertain to teaching Pilates to young people, and identifies the "Magic Window" (ages 9 to 13) as a developmental stage that is particularly favorable for introducing the pedagogy of Pilates.

References

Emmons RA, King LA., 1988. Conflict among personal strivings: immediate and long-term implications for psychological and physical well-being. *Journal of Personality and Social Psychology.* 54(6):1040-8

Ickes, D., 2006. Pilates for Children and Adolescents Workshop

Kraus, S.J., 2002. *Psychological Foundations of Success: A Harvard-Trained Scientist Separates the Science of Success From Self-Help Snake Oil.* San Francisco, Change Planet Press

National Academy of Sports Medicine, 2012. *Youth Exercise Specialist Manual.* Assessment Technologies Institute, LLC

National Prevention, Health Promotion and Public Health Council, 2010. Annual Status Report, July 1, [online] Available at: http://www.surgeongeneral.gov/initiatives/prevention/strategy/mental emotional-well being.pdf

Ward, D. S. et al., 2007. *Physical activity interventions in children and adolescents.* Champaign, IL:Human Kinetics

"Contrology is designed to give you suppleness, natural grace, and skill that will be un-mistakably reflected in the way you walk, in the way you play, and in the way you work."

(Pilates, 1945)

Chapter 3
The Magic Window

The term "Magic Window" originated in the early years of the PMA's efforts to bring Pilates to children. Defining "children and adolescents" as encompassing the ages from 5 to 18, the PMA began by looking at age groups within that range as they reflect specific stages of development. The goal was to identify age groups that would respond well to the neuromuscular nature of Pilates training. In reviewing research in the areas of motor learning, cognitive development and habit formation, one specific age segment appeared to have the most positive long-term outcomes from participating in exercises that integrated the body and mind. This segment, reflecting ages 9 to 13, was named the Magic Window.

The PMA targeted this age group to establish a starting point for Pilates instructors interested in teaching Pilates to children. This particular group was selected because their levels of motor and cognitive development were considered appropriate for participation in a structured exercise program. Selecting an age group where research had (1) established data showing positive outcomes related to physical activity and (2) demonstrated a correlation between physical activity levels and future health benefits increased the feasibility of comparing outcomes from Pilates programs with current studies on physical and cognitive development.

Mind–body Integration

It is during the Magic Window that a concerted effort to highlight mind–body integration exercises can have long-term benefits for young people. Mind–body exercise, the hallmark of Pilates, requires concentration, coordination, and mental awareness to use the body effectively and efficiently as a unified whole. Though this integration applies to all ages and stages of development, it manifests differently during early childhood, middle childhood, and adolescence. An awareness of the developmental changes occurring during these stages of growth is valuable for the preparation and structure of class content.

Early Childhood (Ages 2 - 6)

Early childhood activity is characterized by spontaneous physical expression and play. At this time, there is no perceived distinction between body and mind, which work together as a harmonious unit (Reilly, 1974). The need to be autonomous dominates children's psychosocial development during early childhood, as they are determined to make their own decisions and be independent. According to Erik Erikson's Stages of Psychosocial Development (available online: http://psychology.about.com/library/bl_psychosocial_summary.htm), children need to develop a sense of personal control over physical skills and a sense of independence. Success leads to feelings of autonomy. During this phase, children are able to follow simple rules and understand the relationships between behaviors and feelings. (Solomon and O'Brien, 2011)

Middle Childhood (Ages 7–11)
and Early Adolescence (Ages 12–14)

The transition to middle childhood marks the beginning of more structured and organized play, in addition to balance and coordination function at a higher level. Young people at this stage begin to think abstractly. For example, they are able to envision the outcome of an action without actually doing it.

Middle childhood is a time when children experience a wide range of changes both physically and emotionally (Conger and Galambos 1997). Children encounter new social and academic demands. Success leads to a sense of competence. They become eager to please others and begin to internalize rules, by applying them to themselves, and judge their actions against set standards of behavior.

Developmental psychologists identify certain features of children in this period of development, such as:

- being less self-centered
- being able to recognize ideas or viewpoints that differ from their own
- being able to identify differences and similarities when comparing objects
- the ability to use simple logical thinking to arrive at a conclusion
- the ability to consider multiple aspects of a given situation rather than just one
- the ability to recognize individual objects or pieces as parts of a whole
  (Santrock, 2008)

Adolescence (Ages 12–18)

During this stage of development, young people tend to externalize their own feelings, assuming, for example, that something that bothers or concerns them has the same effect on other people. This tendency can lead to self-consciousness and egocentrism. The use of positive language when teaching this group is extremely important as a means of supporting their development.

Erikson described this stage of development as one where young people struggle to define their identity. The main developmental thrust for adolescents is to develop an acceptable and coherent identity, by combining past experiences with future expectations. They begin to understand themselves based on who they have been and who they hope to be.

The awareness that their bodies and minds can work in harmony creates a basis for managing stress and facing the challenges that adult life can bring. If adolescents are encouraged to learn and experience this mind-body harmony, they may become mindful, present, and aware as they grow and develop into young adults.

Natural Exercises

Joseph Pilates recommended that students "concentrate on the formation of only good habits" and avoid "superficial mechanical exercise which lacks mental concentration," as it may lead to "false conceptions and conclusions in adult life" (Pilates, 1934). To promote optimal health, he encouraged students to learn how to breathe correctly, to understand "correct carriage of the body" (posture) and to practice "natural exercise" (functional movement). Pilates defined natural exercises as those "calculated by Mother Nature to develop her children normally", such as walking, running, jumping, tumbling, climbing, and wrestling. He considered children in the industrialized world to be living in an artificial environment, and believed that they would require a "special course in mind-body training" in order to "consciously control their bodily movements until the good habits formed become subconscious routine acts."

Pilates offers an opportunity to perform natural exercises such as Rolling Back (sometimes called "Rolling Like a Ball") and The Seal, which combine integrated movement with body awareness in an enjoyable activity.

Adaptations to Resistance Training

Resistance training is defined as the use of progressive exercise to increase a person's ability to exert or resist force, through a variety of training modalities used to overload the muscles (Faigenbaum, 1998; Boyce, 2006). During the Magic Window, the body adapts to resistance training via both neural (increased motor recruitment) and biochemical (muscle hypertrophy) mechanisms. Strength gains come predominantly from neural adaptations rather than size changes in the muscle tissue. The theory behind this is that higher levels of sex hormones activate the neural circuits within the body (Romeo, 2003). Prior to the Magic Window, neural mechanisms and motors skills are not fully developed. As a result, balance, coordination and whole body movement can be challenging. The Magic Window is the ideal time to use awareness of mind-body connections to enhance movement capabilities for daily activities, sports, and exercise in general.

After puberty, muscle hypertrophy (increase in the size of muscles) occurs due to changes in testosterone levels (Rowland, 2005). Figure 3.1 shows that neural development increases rapidly in children from birth to age 12, *reaching maturation between the ages of 8 and 12, which roughly correlates with the Magic Window target group, ages 9 to 13*. In the graph, skeletal growth progresses steadily, with a marked increase from ages 8 to 16. Muscular development is steady and minimal by comparison until ages 14 to 20 (Anderson and Twist, 2005).

The Magic Window has been highlighted in the graph in blue to show that children between the ages of 8 and 12 are close to full neurological maturity. However, significant physiological changes are yet to come.

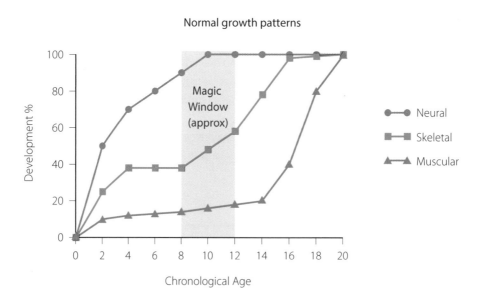

Figure 3.1. Graph data from trainability of children by Anderson and Twist, 2005

Long-term Outcomes

Well-applied physical exercise develops a child's body and mind, and positively influences their self-perception. Teaching Pilates to children in the Magic Window age group holds great promise for promoting their long-term health and achievement. Providing good movement education and physical awareness at this time fosters important skills for navigating puberty, which is just around the corner.

Conclusion

The Magic Window age range (ages 9 to 13) has been identified as the ideal time to introduce young people to Pilates. For the purposes of teaching Pilates to young people, it is useful to be aware of the developmental changes young people undergo in the stages of early childhood, middle childhood, and adolescence. As young people in the Magic Window are close to full neurological maturity, this age range represents a developmental stage where movement skills can be incorporated and mastered so as to create positive habits that can be carried into adulthood. At this time, young people's motor and cognitive skills are mature enough to allow them to follow the Pilates movement principles and understand their importance in supporting whole body health.

Chapter 4 will explore fundamental teaching practices and considerations that support the teacher's thinking and strategy in presenting a Pilates program for young people.

References

Anderson, G. S., Twist, P., 2005. Trainability of children. *IDEA Fitness Journal,* March

Boyce, P., 2006. *Orthopaedic Physical Therapy Secrets,* 2nd ed. St Louis: Mosby

Conger J. J., Galambos N. L., 1997. *Adolescence and youth: psychological development in a changing world.* 5th ed. New York: Longman

Erikson, Erik H., 1959. *Identity and the Life Cycle.* New York: International Universities Press

Erikson, Erik H., 1968. *Identity, Youth and Crisis.* New York: Norton

Faigenbaum, A.D., Bradley D.F., 1998. Strength training for the young athlete. *Orthopedic Physical Therapy Clin N Am.* 7, 67-90.

Pilates, J. H., 1934. *Your Health.* Reprinted in: A Pilates' primer: The millennium edition. Incline Village, NV: Presentation Dynamics Inc.

Reilly, M., 1974. *Play as exploratory learning.* London: Sage Publications

Romeo, R.D., 2003. Puberty: a period of both organizational and activational effects of steroid hormones on neurobehavioural development. *Journal of Neuroendocrinology.* 15(12):1185-92. Laboratory of Neuroendocrinology, Rockefeller University

Rowland, T. W., 2005. *Children's exercise physiology.* Champaign, IL: Human Kinetics

Santrock, J.W., 2008. *Life-Span Development,* 12th ed. New York: McGraw-Hill Humanities

Solomon, J., O'Brien, J., 2011. *Pediatric Skills for Occupational Therapy Assistants,* 3rd ed. St Louis: Mosby

"Contrology develops the body uniformly, corrects wrong postures, restores physical vitality, invigorates the mind, and elevates the spirit." (Pilates, 1945)

Chapter 4
Teaching Practice and Considerations

This chapter introduces a range of practical matters and educational strategies, the purpose of which is to inform the Pilates teacher's thinking and planning. A thorough consideration of these topics will empower the Pilates teacher to go forward into the work with insight and a broad perspective on working with young people.

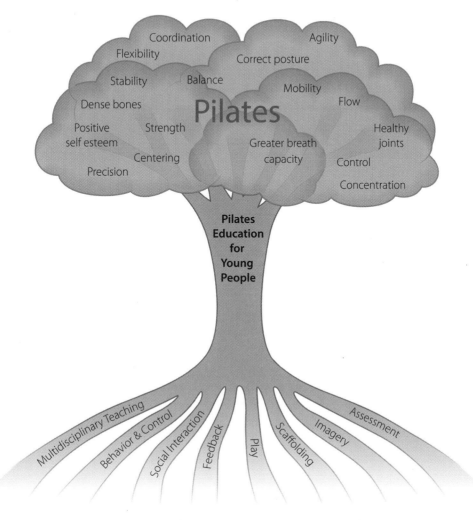

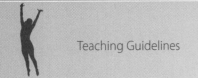

Approaching Your Learners

Young People as Learners

Teaching Pilates to children and adolescents involves much more than knowledge of the Pilates exercises. To teach with success for this specific population of learners, the teacher must make effective decisions about what Pilates content is going to be taught as well as *how* the content will be taught. It is important to remember that children and adolescents are not adults. Their past experiences, cognitively and physiologically, are different from those of an adult, resulting in a different kind of learning experience.

Example:

In the case of adults, the execution of Pilates exercises will generally be different for a client with a strong past movement background, who leads an active life, than for a client with no past movement background, who leads a sedentary life. These clients' past and present experiences differ from one another, resulting in a difference in their learning experience. This disparity in experience is similar to the difference between the young and adult learner.

> *"A teacher of young children must be aware of the limitations of a child's growing body, lack of motor learning experiences, and immature perceptual and cognitive skills on skill acquisition and allow a child to enjoy the experience of moving and exploration, while offering external guidance, instruction and evaluation"* (Kimmerle and Cote-Laurence, 2003). See Mind-Body Integration section of Magic Window chapter 3.

Young people's bodies and brains are growing and developing rapidly. Their perception, proprioception and cognition are evolving. A Pilates teacher must transmit the material given to a child or adolescent in a way that is fun, creative and developmentally appropriate. In doing so, it is useful for the teacher to have a clear intent regarding the learning objectives they would like to achieve.

Students' Involvement with Movement – A Spectrum

Pilates teachers working with young people will sometimes find themselves teaching students whose interest in or involvement with movement is moderate or low. For example, such students may have a strong interest in intellectual pursuits and academics, and little interest in activities that require physical skills, such as sports or dance. The lack of engagement with movement may also be a reflection of a lack of opportunity. Alternatively, teachers will also encounter young people who are involved in pursuits requiring highly developed movement skills at a pre-professional level in, for example, sports, dance, or gymnastics. As a result, the focus of the teaching should be considered and adapted to address this range of students. Teachers may need to adapt the class to focus on "process", "product", or a combination of both.

Focus on "process" (experience and development)

For students with a moderate to low level of involvement in movement activities, the teacher might focus on providing the students with Pilates movement experiences that enhance body awareness, mind-body integration, and relaxation, focus and concentration through breathing practice. The improvements in overall strength, balance and flexibility that result from Pilates exercise and that benefit all people, will definitely benefit young people with a limited involvement in movement. Such students could consider how to apply what they learn in Pilates class to movement in their daily activities outside of the Pilates classroom.

Focus on "product" (skill and execution)

For students engaged in developing advanced movement skills for activities such as gymnastics, ice-skating or ballet, the teacher might add to the "process" approach mentioned above and put additional emphasis on "product"; in other words, how well the Pilates movements are being performed. Such students can use Pilates exercise to help them develop precise, sophisticated physical skills required for their sports or dance activities, at a pre-professional level.

Combining focuses on "process" and "product"

Depending on the makeup of the class, the teacher can weight the activities more toward "process" or "product". Ultimately, they do go hand in hand.

Pilates teachers should consider the makeup of their student group, and determine the most appropriate and helpful teaching focus.

(The analysis above is adapted from Jacqueline Smith-Autard's discussion of teaching models in her book, *The Art of Dance Education*, 1994.)

Know Your Learner

It is well known that people learn and process information in a variety of ways. According to Fleming and Mills' VARK model, the primary sensory modalities used for learning information are: Visual (V), Aural (A), Read/Write (R), and Kinesthetic (K). Human life is multi-modal, and these modalities do overlap. Generally speaking, students may show a preference for *visual learning* (preference for the visual depiction of information), *auditory learning* (a person learns through listening and speaking) *read/write learning* (preference for information displayed as words), or *kinesthetic learning* (learning through personal experience or practice).

A Pilates teacher should assess the learning styles of their students, and adapt their teaching approach, wherever possible, to the ways in which their students learn best. The teacher might demonstrate an exercise or make use of a mirror for feedback for a visual learner, give descriptive cues with rhythms for an auditory learner, or adjust the body positioning of a kinesthetic learner.

With regard to kinesthetic learners, it must be remembered that when teaching Pilates to children and adolescents there will be circumstances where the teacher is not allowed to touch their students, because of a teaching environment's established policies. In these conditions, the teacher will need to use creativity when giving feedback to kinesthetic learners.

Example: *The Hundred*
(using the wall as a prop)

If the teacher is asking the students to hold their legs at a certain height when performing the exercise (e.g., 12 inches off the ground), the teacher could have the students position their feet an inch away from the wall. In this way, if the students' legs drop below 12 inches, they will feel their feet touch the wall, giving them feedback on whether or not they are maintaining the position.

Example: *The One Leg Kick*
(the student uses their own touch for feedback)

If the teacher is asking the students to recognize if they are maintaining their pelvic stability while executing the exercise, the teacher could have the students place their hands underneath their hipbones (ASIS bones) to feel if their pelvis is rotating while alternating leg kicks.

Teaching Procedures

Classroom Environment and Equipment

Pilates can be taught in many environments, from Pilates, ballet, or exercise studios to many kinds of educational settings. Pilates teachers working in schools may be required to teach in a classroom, on a stage, in a gym, on a playing field, or other locations within the school. In these cases, teachers should consider what limitations the setting provides and what can be used or altered in the setting to create an optimal learning environment for Pilates.

Setup

It is advisable to have the classroom pre-set before the start of class, with all materials and props in place. It may be appropriate to have a special student helper assist in pre-setting the classroom. If so, the teacher can have students take turns being the helper, in order to give everyone a chance to participate.

When positioning the mats, the teacher can arrange the mats in a variety of ways to suit how their lesson will be conducted. For example, mats can be arranged by rows, staggered, mirrored, or in a circle. Mats should be a minimum of ¾ of an inch thick, for the protection of the spine and head. If mats are not readily available or are not in the budget, the teacher can explore the possibility of having them donated by a mat manufacturer or a Pilates conference. Towels or carpet squares can also be used in place of mats, but will need to be at least ¾ of an inch thick. If towels or carpet squares are to be used, they can be doubled or folded to achieve the appropriate thickness.

If mirrors are available, the teacher should consider whether or not to use mirrors as a tool. The teacher should evaluate whether it would be useful for their students to use mirrors to provide feedback on exercise performance, or whether mirrors would cause unwanted distractions. If the latter is the case, the students can do their class facing away from the mirrors.

In working with young people, simple props may be helpful for certain kinds of exercises. If props are not available, the teacher may be able to provide or create their own inexpensive props.

Examples of inexpensive props:

- A pinwheel, to recreate the Pilates Breath Exerciser.
- Large rubber bands, to be used as the Pilates Toe Exerciser.

Classroom Management

Ratio of adults to students

In planning the work, the teacher must determine how many students will be in the class and whether an assistant will be required. It is generally recommended to have a maximum of 10 students per one adult. Even if the class size is small, it is advisable to have a second adult in the classroom if possible. This is helpful with regard to classroom management and emergencies, but it is also helpful with regard to liability. A second adult can provide verification of what is and is not happening in the classroom. The second adult may be the regular classroom teacher, a teacher's aide, or a parent.

Entering and leaving the classroom

The teacher will need to establish a safe, orderly and effective way to get students in and out of the classroom space. To maintain order and safety, it is not advisable to have all the students enter and exit at once. An entrance and exit strategy should be planned in advance.

The teacher should consider whether to have the students enter one at a time, in a line, or in small groups. An example of the latter might be to have students enter or exit by their birthday months, or by the first letter of their last names.

The teacher should also choose whether the students will begin the class seated or standing. With the Early Childhood and Magic Window age groups, it is advisable to have the students begin the class seated, to prevent unnecessary movement.

Focus Exercise

At the beginning of class, it may at times be appropriate to use a focus exercise to help center the students and bring their attention to the present. *Passing the Imaginary Ball* is a good example of a focus exercise. The exercise is done with the students standing in a circle. (Sitting is advised when first doing this exercise with the Early Childhood and Magic Window age groups.) The teacher creatively passes an imaginary ball to the student next to them (for example, passing the ball as if it is extremely heavy, or juggling the ball, imagining that it is a hot potato). The ball is passed around the circle creatively from student to student until it returns to the teacher. While the ball is being passed, the teacher "sportscasts", giving a play-by-play description of every action (as in, "Clara is slowly rolling ball from one arm across her shoulders, and now the ball is accelerating quickly down her other arm").

This kind of focus exercise is useful for developing creativity in students, defining anatomical landmarks of the body, and establishing a movement vocabulary, while maintaining focus on the ball throughout the exercise. Before beginning the exercise, it is helpful for the teacher to give some examples of how the ball can be passed, to spark the students' imagination.

Breathing awareness exercises are also very helpful for creating focus and concentration in students.

Planning the Lesson

It is important for the teacher to plan and structure the lessons in advance, with a clear goal for what will be achieved by the end of each class, as well as by the end of the sequence of classes. The following is a list of suggested components of an individual class:

- Entering the class space
- A focus exercise
- A warm-up
- The body of the lesson
- Cool down
- Leaving the class space

(See Chapter 10, *Curriculum for Schools*, for more information on lesson planning.)

Teaching Practice

This section discusses important strategies and considerations for the classroom work itself. This subject matter will be helpful to Pilates teachers who have not worked with young people in the past.

Imagery

"Imagery", as discussed here, refers to mental pictures or images. As a teaching tool, it involves the use of vivid or figurative language to represent objects, actions, or ideas. "Images are teaching cues to help to prepare, initiate and execute movements properly. Imagery is the use of a mental picture to accomplish a physical task with greater ease and efficiency of motion"(Barnett, 2010).

Example: *The Spine Stretch*

When having a student roll up through their spine, one vertebra at a time, a teacher might say, "Imagine that you are stringing a pearl necklace. As you roll up through your spine, string one pearl on top of another." For young children, a teacher might suggest that they imagine stacking building blocks one on top of another.

> *"The image should be suited to the clients' image vocabulary, so that he or she can relate to the image and infer meaning." (Isacowitz, 2006)*

In working with young people, it is helpful to select vivid, easily graspable images, and to exemplify those images throughout the lesson. To use imagery effectively, it is important to be clear, descriptive and deliberate with word choice, and to weave chosen words and images into themes that can be built upon.

Example: *Snake Lesson*

(See *Sample Lesson Plans* in Chapter 10, *Curriculum for Schools*)

The teacher presents a wooden toy snake, and asks the students to suggest words describing how the snake moves and sounds, and to then incorporate the movements implied by those words into their own bodies, creating a movement vocabulary. Incorporating the snake vernacular and movements into the various components of the lesson carries the theme of the Snake forward:

- Entrance Strategy- Students make a single file line, then weave that line into the classroom like a snake "slithering".
- Warm-up (Snake Breath)- Breathing in and out, with an extended "hissing" on the exhalation.

- Use of images and words like "coil", "undulate", and "ripple" during the Pilates exercises. For example, in Rolling Back, keeping the body in a tight snake "coil" while rolling back and forth.
- Cool Down- Wiggling different anatomical landmarks of the body, imitating a snake "squirming".

Scaffolding

"Scaffolding" is a term that refers to a learning process where a teacher provides specific supports or aids to learning when concepts and skills are first being introduced to students. Such supports are gradually removed as students assimilate the new material. As a metaphor for the concept of scaffolding in teaching, it is helpful to think of the scaffolding used in the construction of a new building. In building construction, scaffolding is used as a support for people and materials during the building process.

In teaching Pilates, a good example of scaffolding would be "deconstructing" an exercise. If a student has difficulty executing an exercise, the teacher might break down the skills involved so that the student can master each skill separately. Later, by combining the skills, the student can do the original exercise with success.

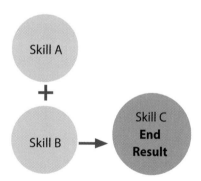

Example: The *One Leg Stretch*
A. The student learns and masters the choreography of the arms.
B. The student learns and masters the choreography of the legs.
C. The student combines the choreography of the arms and legs.

Props

The use of props is another example of scaffolding in Pilates. Props can be used to assist with an exercise or concept, and can provide feedback to the student.

Example 1: *The Roll-Up*

Use a towel or mat as a prop. If a student has trouble rolling up, the teacher can suggest using a towel or mat to assist the movement. The student lies on the towel or mat, reaches back and grasps the end corners of the towel or mat, and then pulls on the ends to assist them in rolling up.

Example 2: *Rolling Back*

Use a ball as a prop. The student places a ball between their torso and legs and squeezes the ball, with equal pressure from the upper and lower body, as they roll back and forth. The squeezing of the ball helps to reinforce the idea of using the body as a compact ball, and provides feedback to the student as to whether they are using more upper body or lower body pressure when rolling.

Example 3: *The Hundred, The One Leg Stretch, or The Double Leg Stretch*

Use a ball or a rubber ducky. The student balances the ball or rubber ducky on their navel when performing these exercises, while engaging their transverse abdominal muscles. If the student doesn't engage these muscles properly, the ball will roll off or the rubber ducky will rise.

If the teacher's budget doesn't allow for the kinds of props described above, objects that are already in the classroom can be used in scaffolding.

Example 4: *The Hundred or The Teaser*

Use the wall to assist the movement.

Students can bring their feet against the wall for support in exercises like The Hundred and The Teaser.

Multidisciplinary Teaching

A Pilates teacher working with young people has the opportunity to make their classes multidisciplinary, tying in other subjects such as science, reading, or math. This can potentially make Pilates education more valuable to school administrators, in linking it with other areas of study.

Note

For more detailed explanations of the examples below, see *Sample Lesson Plans* in Chapter 10, *Curriculum for Schools.*

Example: Early Childhood –*The Snake Lesson*
(Vocabulary)

In exploring the ways that a snake moves, children will learn vocabulary words that describe a range of snake-like behaviors, such as "wiggle", "slither", or "hiss".

Example: Middle Childhood – *The Three-Movement Circus*
(Human Physiology)

By exploring how movement occurs in three dimensions (in the sagittal, coronal and transverse planes), students will be able to identify the three dimensions and give examples of movement in each dimension.

Example: Adolescence – *Moving from the Center Out*
(Astronomy)

The lesson plan draws parallels between how the planets of the solar system rotate around the sun and how the peripheral body parts extend from and relate to the core of the body.

Behavior and Control

Behavior

Appropriate behavior in students is very important in order to maintain a safe, healthy, and efficient learning environment. Appropriate behavior is a reflection of mutual trust and respect, not only within the student/teacher relationship, but also within the relationship between the students. It involves cooperation and a respect for the rules of the classroom culture. When teaching a new group of children or adolescents it is very important to establish, at the outset, what the rules of the classroom are. Students must learn that there are consequences for their actions, including the breaking of rules, and that there are benefits to appropriate behavior.

Control

The teacher must determine how much control they are going to exercise, and how much independence they are going to allow the students. Control can be categorized as High, Medium and Low.

In a **High Control** environment, the teacher directs the classroom activity using a "command" form of teaching. The teacher is in charge, and students must follow their directions. The student has very little input in decision-making.

In **Medium Control**, the teacher assigns tasks, and allows the students to work independently whenever possible. Students have some input in decision-making, though the teacher makes the final decisions.

Low Control gives students a greater degree of independence. The teacher may choose to use a "reciprocal" learning approach. Reciprocal learning involves students explaining their learning to other students, and taking turns acting as the teacher. Students are encouraged to evaluate their execution of a task. The teacher acts as a facilitator, and students play a more direct role in decision-making.

The teacher must decide which type of control will work best for the population of students they are working with. When entering a teaching environment that already has an established code of discipline, it is advisable for the teacher to adapt to that environment's approach, even if it is not what the teacher prefers. Within any teaching environment, there may be times when the students become unfocused or chaotic, and it is helpful for teachers to have ways of re-focusing the class. Using "call and response" is a quick and effective way of regaining control of the group.

Example

The teacher makes a game out of "call and response". The teacher instructs the students that when he or she performs a specific rhythmic clapping phrase, the students must respond with their own rhythmic clapping phrase—as in:

The Call (Teacher): Clap, Clap __ Clap, Clap, Clap.

The Response (Students): Clap, Clap __ Clap, Clap.

The "call and response" stops unfocused activity and noise. Clapping involves using the body- in this case, the hands; students concentrate on clapping with their hands instead of walking, running, or jumping. Clapping creates a sound; students concentrate on creating the rhythm of the clap instead of speaking or vocalizing. This technique allows the teacher to regain control without raising their voice.

Keep it moving

It is important to remember that a young person's attention span is shorter than an adult's. Therefore, it is advisable to keep the pace of the class moving, and to vary the activities. Keeping the class moving also helps to prevent students from becoming bored or restless, or losing focus.

Assessment and Feedback

Assessment

Assessment as used in this manual, refers to various ways in which a teacher can measure or evaluate students' progress and success with the work. Assessment is both for the students' and the teacher's benefit, and is used to ascertain whether or not the desired learning objectives are being achieved. It provides accountability for both students and teachers, encourages the teacher to look at each student and evaluate their progress, and provides data that allows for future development and planning of programming.

Forms of Assessment		
Observation	*Journals*	*Demonstrations*
Class Discussion	*Essays*	*Quizzes or Tests*
Homework	*Performance Tasks*	*Rubrics*
Exit Slips	*Exhibitions*	*Self or Peer Evaluation*

The following are examples of how the forms of assessment listed above can be used in the teaching of Pilates.

Example: Class Discussion

"What is Pilates, and what/who is it good for?"

Example: Essay

Students are asked to write an essay about Joseph Pilates and his work.

Example: Exit Slip

Before exiting the classroom, students are asked to write, and hand in, answers to questions such as:

- "At what moment in class today did you feel the most engaged with what was happening?"
- "What action that anyone (instructor or participant) took in class today did you find most affirming or helpful?"
- Use an "I" statement about class today (e.g. "I learned...", "I felt..." "I imagined...", "I am...")

Feedback

Feedback is an ongoing and necessary component of teaching. The teacher is responsible for providing relevant feedback to the students for their development and progress. Feedback from the teacher can help students correct errors and motivate them to continue to practice or perform. It can be both positive and corrective. Positive feedback helps to motivate students, and reinforces correct performance; corrective feedback helps students to identify and correct specific errors. In giving feedback, it is important not to overwhelm the students with corrections. There is a limit to students' memory and attention capacity. When a student is new to an experience, one correction is generally enough, and it should be directed to the most important priorities of the activity that the students are practicing. This one correction may be repeated, to reinforce it. Ideally, the teacher should foster self-awareness in students, so that they can learn to correct themselves.

Educational Environments and Standards

Educational Environments

Possible environments where a Pilates program may be implemented include:

State-funded: public and charter schools

Most schools that are funded by public money require a curriculum to be presented and approved by school administrators, in order for a new program to be implemented. A curriculum outlines the planned interaction of students with course content, materials and resources, and the processes for evaluating whether or not the educational objectives have been met. (See Chapter 10, *Curriculum for Schools*)

If it is not feasible for the school in question to accept a Pilates curriculum, the teacher might find that there is more flexibility in after-school programs or outreach programs based at the school.

Fee-paying: private and parochial schools

In most cases, fee-paying schools are not subject to the same rules and regulations as state-funded schools, and it can be easier for them to accept new programs such as Pilates. Private schools (fee paying) will generally have fewer restrictions and more access to funding sources, and may provide better opportunities for implementation of a Pilates program.

Other facilities

Other environments where a Pilates program for young people might be held include Pilates, dance, or martial arts studios, recreation centers, summer camps, or sport facilities. It is usually easier to implement a Pilates program for young people in these types of settings than in a school setting, as there may be fewer and more flexible decision-makers involved.

Gender-Segregated Environments

In Pilates teaching, the decision to have a coed class or a gender-segregated class will not always be made by the teacher. A Pilates teacher should recognize that certain settings will require the students to be separated by gender. This may be based on various factors, such as age and maturity, religious beliefs, or the culture or rules of the teaching environment.

Educational Standards

Pilates teachers should strongly consider addressing established standards for physical education in their teaching. Standards provide educators with guidelines for what students should know and be able to do. Pilates teachers should refer to standards in developing curriculums, and in assessing whether students are achieving the prescribed learning objectives.

In the US, the National Association for Sports and Physical Education (NASPE) Standards are a useful guide for working in schools. For those working in the dance education community, the National Dance Education Organization (NDEO) Standards are useful as well. A Pilates teacher's proposed curriculum should include information on physical education or dance education standards, and show how their proposed Pilates class will address those standards.

See: National Association for Sports and Physical Education (NASPE)
www.aahperd.org/naspe/standards/nationalstandards/pestandards.cfm
National Dance Education Organization (NDEO) www.ndeo.org.

Conclusion

Through an awareness of young people's needs as learners, and a clear understanding of educational strategies, teachers can confidently undertake the inspiring opportunity to further Joseph Pilates' vision by bringing this remarkable work to younger generations.

Chapter 5, the concluding chapter of the Teaching Guidelines section of this book, discusses administrative procedures, safety and matters of ethics and professionalism.

References

Isacowitz, R., 2006. *Pilates.* Champaign, IL: Human Kinetics

Kimmerle, M., Cote-Laurence, P., 2003. *Teaching dance skills: A motor learning and development approach.* Andover, NJ: J. Michael Ryan Publishing

Smith-Autard, J. M., 1994. *The art of dance in education.* London, UK: Bloomsbury Publishing Plc.

The Vark Categories. (n.d.), [online] Available at:
    http://www.vark-learn.com/english/page.asp?p=categories

Wiggins, G., McTighe, J., 2006. *Understanding by design: Expanded 2nd ed.* Upper Saddle River, NJ: Pearson Merrill Prentice Hall

"With body, mind and spirit functioning perfectly as a coordinated whole, what else could reasonably be expected other than an active, alert, disciplined person?"

(Pilates, 1945)

Chapter 5
General Procedures, Safety, and Professionalism

This chapter discusses important procedures within the teaching facility, matters of safety, and professionalism as they apply to teaching Pilates to young people.

The opening section outlines a range of procedures, administrative forms, and permissions that the Pilates teacher should be aware of and may need to put in place, depending on the teaching environment.

General Procedures

1. Liability insurance

a. **General and Professional Liability Insurance**. This is essential for all Pilates teachers.

b. **Abuse and Molestation Coverage**. Teachers should consider whether they want to also carry Abuse and Molestation coverage. If the teacher makes the decision to forgo sexual abuse and molestation coverage, they will be responsible in the event of a charge, for providing funds for their own defense, as well as any amount awarded against them, even if the charge is groundless. If the teacher does elect to purchase abuse and molestation coverage, they should consider whether or not to choose a policy that includes image restoration as a policy benefit. The PMA recommends seeking legal advice for any questions regarding this subject.

2. Administrative forms

In the case of schools and other institutional settings, it is the Pilates teacher's responsibility to be familiar with the institution's policies and procedures, including those regarding any administrative forms.

When the teacher is working privately, the administrative forms listed below are essential.

Ultimately, it is the Pilates teacher's responsibility to consult with their legal advisor about applicable forms and their content.

a. **Waiver of Liability and Informed Consent Release**

For young people under 18, a waiver of liability and informed consent release should be signed by each student's parent or guardian. This does not guarantee freedom from liability. The precise contents of the form may vary from setting to setting. It is the responsibility of the teacher and facility owner to verify, through their legal advisor and/or insurance company, which inclusions and restrictions may apply.

b. **Health and Medical History Intake**

It is standard procedure to have a health and medical history intake form for each student. For students under the age of 18, the form should be filled out by a parent or guardian.

c. **Media/Photography Release**

In the case of children being photographed, release forms must be signed by a parent or guardian. These should be filled out prior to any photos being taken to protect the teacher and the facility from liability.

d. **Incident Report**

An incident report form should be used to document any incident that causes the teacher concern. This form should include:

- A description of the incident by the teacher.
- Statements from any witnesses, as well as their contact information.

3. Fingerprinting, safety classes and background check

In schools and community centers, teachers are often required to be fingerprinted, to undergo police background checks and to take special safety classes. Individual institutions will specify their policies regarding these procedures.

4. First aid

a. In most cases, educational institutions and teaching facilities have established protocols regarding first aid, which the teacher is required to follow.

b. If there is a nurse on-site, establishing a chain of communication and procedural guidelines will assist the teacher in understanding their role in the event of an emergency or injury.

c. A first aid kit should be available on-site. Depending on the specific circumstances or teaching environment, it may be the teacher's responsibility to provide the kit.

d. Individual institutions and facilities may require teachers to have first aid training in cardiopulmonary resuscitation (CPR) or automated external defibrillator use (AED). Courses in children's first aid are available, and many US states require teachers to be CPR-certified when working with children.

e. In case of emergency, teachers must have contact details for the parent or guardian of each child, as well as information about any allergies or medical conditions. (Typically, this information will appear on the health intake form.)

5. **Disaster preparedness**

   Protocols for natural disasters, such as earthquakes, tornados, or hurricanes, should be in place where applicable.

6. **Procedure with regard to incidents**

   In the event of an incident, the Incident Report referenced in 2.d. above should be completed, and a protocol for managing the remainder of the class should be in place.

Safety

Teachers must be aware that they are responsible for safety within the teaching environment, and as such, basic safety procedures should be established and followed. If the teaching facility already has safety procedures in place, the teacher must be aware of them and observe them. If the teaching facility has no such procedures in place, or if the procedures in place are inadequate, it is the teacher's responsibility to establish and implement sufficient safety protocols.

The following is a basic list of safety precautions:

- Determine how many students will be in the class and if an assistant will be required. It is generally recommended to have a maximum of 10 students per one adult. Even if the class size is small, it is advisable to have a second adult in the classroom if possible. This is helpful with regard to classroom management and emergencies, but it is also helpful with regard to liability. A second adult can provide verification of what is and is not happening in the classroom. The second adult may be the regular classroom teacher, a teacher's aide, or a parent.

- The safety of the students during class is the teacher's responsibility, unless expressly stated otherwise. The students' safety after class is also the teacher's responsibility, until they are picked up by a parent or guardian.

- All exercises should be performed on a mat of a minimum thickness of ¾ of an inch, for protection of the spine and head. Failure to use mats of the appropriate thickness may cause injury.

- Adequate floor space for each student must be provided. Each student should have a space on the floor equal to a 5 to 6-foot square. One way to test whether the students have adequate floor space is to ask them while lying on the mat to make an X with their bodies or pretend to make "snow angels". If a student touches another student while performing these tasks, they are too close to one another.

- Fatigue is an important consideration for safety and proper performance of the exercises. If the student appears fatigued, distressed, flushed, or pale, there are several options to consider:
  - Modify the movement.
  - Have the student assume a rest position:
    - Lie supine, hugging the knees to the chest.
    - Assume Child's Pose.
- Proper hydration is important for all young people. Children thermoregulate differently from adults in both hot and cold climates, and they require more water than adults and frequent breaks.
- Teachers should be mindful and attentive to changes in students' complexion, increased heart rate, profuse sweating, or any other indications that they are having an adverse response to exercise. If any of these conditions are observed, the teacher should cease the exercise immediately and attend to the child.
- Pain is an immediate indication to STOP activity. Students should be told that if they experience any form of pain, they must immediately stop the exercise and inform the teacher.
  - If there is a nurse on staff, the student should be escorted to the nurse (or the nurse should be called to the scene) for a proper medical assessment.
  - An incident report must be filled out for any incidence of pain or discomfort which causes the student to stop the exercise and seek medical attention.
  - If there is no nurse on staff, the student should be taken aside to rest and the teacher must complete a report. The teacher must decide if further action needs to be taken.
- Students should be made aware that practicing Pilates is not a competition. They should be encouraged to work at their own level, and should be familiar with the symptoms of fatigue and how to rest in an appropriate position.
- Proper attire for participation should be worn. Clothing that is too loose or too tight should be avoided. Overly loose clothing obscures the teacher's view of the student's body, and may be an impediment to movement. Clothing that is too tight may restrict breathing. It is advisable to remove jewelry and watches, which may be a distraction, may cause injury, or may be damaged.
- Rolling exercises (on the back) should always stop at the shoulder area or upper back. Students should be instructed to avoid rolling onto their necks or heads.

- As stated in Chapter 1, *programming should avoid inversion exercises* like The Jack-Knife and The Roll-Over during the middle teen years, as these exercises load the spine during a time when growth plate fusion is still occurring. *All contraindicated exercises for young people have been excluded from this manual.*

- Safety procedures should include a protocol for what to do in the event of an incident.

The following is a brief overview of basic procedure for incidents:

1) Identify the problem.
2) Instruct the student involved in the incident to stop the activity.
3) Identify two students to go and get help.
4) If the student involved is conscious and coherent, determine the need for emergency medical care (call emergency services), and contact the student's parent(s) or guardian.
5) If appropriate, administer CPR.
6) Document the incident in detail, using an incident report form.

Code of Ethics

When teaching children and adolescents, the Pilates teacher must demonstrate the highest ethical standards. The PMA's Code of Ethics is attached as an Appendix to this manual, and is a good example of the standards Pilates teachers should adhere to. These ethical codes, however, were written with teaching adults in mind, and the following should be observed when teaching young people:

- Young people must be treated with dignity, and, at all times, proper teacher/student boundaries must be observed. While treating students with kindness and friendliness, remember that the teacher is not the student's personal friend, rather they are an adult in authority.
- The teacher should show tolerance and respect for others, bearing in mind that their own personal beliefs and opinions may be different from those of the child and the child's family.

Scope of Practice

The PMA has established a formal Scope of Practice document for Pilates professionals, which lists actions that fall within the professional role of a Pilates teacher, as well as actions that are beyond that role. The Scope of Practice document is attached as an Appendix to this manual.

Professional Conduct

The professional conduct of a Pilates teacher can be defined as the teacher's behavior within their working environment. The teacher's behavior must be grounded in both the Code of Ethics and Scope of Practice for the profession.

A primary principle that applies to working with children is that the Pilates teacher will do no harm. Professional demeanor should be based in treating children with kindness and approaching the work in a spirit of inspiration and enthusiasm.

It is important for teachers to remember that their conduct in class influences both the outcome of the work and ultimately their students' ability to learn effectively.

The following are some key points to consider with regard to professional conduct in working with young people:

- Dress appropriately.
- Use appropriate and positive language.
- Keep all necessary forms on site and accessible.
- Show respect for students' privacy.

The Pilates Teacher as a Role Model

A Pilates teacher working with young people has an extraordinary opportunity to be a positive role model for their students. Teaching the pedagogy and values of Pilates brings with it the chance to inspire young people to care about their own physical health and well-being, and to learn how these factors can improve their experience of living.

For a young person, learning a physical discipline of this kind builds confidence in their ability to achieve, and helps them to focus, to be more calm, and to have more self-esteem. The role and influence of the teacher are integral to all of this.

As an example to their students, teachers must be aware that their own good grooming and physical fitness are important demonstrations of the values of Pilates, as are good nutrition and adequate rest.

In addition, teachers can make a meaningful and highly valued contribution to their students' lives through embodying these attributes of positive role models:

- Role models live their own values in the world.
- Role models show a commitment to helping and empowering others.
- Role models demonstrate personal effectiveness and the possibility of overcoming obstacles.
- Perhaps most important of all, role models show passion for their work and the ability to inspire others (Price-Mitchell, 2013).

Conclusion

Teaching Pilates to children requires compliance with specific legal and managerial responsibilities, including matters such as liability insurance, proper consent and medical forms, first aid and CPR, and how to respond in the case of an incident. In addition, appropriate safety considerations must be addressed, such as the proper monitoring of students' response to the work and the avoidance of inversion exercises, as well as appropriate class size, mats, and clothing. Finally, as adults teaching children and adolescents, Pilates teachers have a responsibility to realize that young people may model their behavior, and they must therefore demonstrate high standards in the way they present themselves, interact with others, and communicate.

With all of these elements in place, teachers can confidently focus on teaching Pilates.

Reference

Price-Mitchell, M., 2013. *What is a role model, five qualities that matter to teens.* [Online] Available at: www.rootsofaction.com

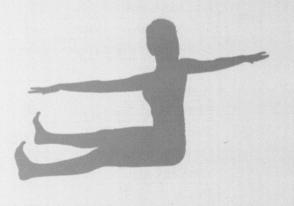

Section Two
The Exercise Chapters

Note 1: Understanding the developmental changes in early childhood, middle childhood and adolescence is essential for designing a safe and effective Pilates program for young people. This manual references Solomon's definitions of the stages and ages of development. As such, please note that there is a degree of overlap in the way that age groupings are identified in subsequent chapters of this text (Solomon, 2011).

Note 2: The following chapters contain a range of Pilates exercises that are appropriate for children and adolescents. All contraindicated exercises have been completely excluded from this manual.

	Children Ages 5 - 8	Children & Adolescents Ages 9 - 13 Magic Window	Adolescents Ages 12 - 18
Chapter 6 - Pre-Pilates Exercises			
Breathing Awareness	✓	✓	✓
Pelvic Awareness	✓	✓	✓
Cervical Awareness	✓	✓	✓
Rib Cage Awareness	✓	✓	✓
Shoulder Girdle Awareness - Supine	✓	✓	✓
Shoulder Girdle Awareness - Prone	✓	✓	✓
Airplane Arms	✓	✓	✓
Sitting - Shrugs	✓	✓	✓
Sitting - Hug a Tree	✓	✓	✓
Standing - Shrugs	✓	✓	✓
Standing - Hug a Tree	✓	✓	✓
Spinal Mobility	✓	✓	✓
The Cat	✓	✓	✓
The Bridge	✓	✓	✓
Hover	✓	✓	✓
Rib Curl	✓	✓	✓
Hip Folds	✓	✓	✓
Toe Taps	✓	✓	✓
Double Knee Drop Side	✓	✓	✓
Chapter 7 - Pilates Exercises for Early Childhood, Ages 5–8			
Imaginary Jump Rope Warm-up	✓	✓	✓
Standing Sequence	✓	✓	✓
Stand to Sit (Transition)	✓	✓	✓
The Hundred (Modified - Kneeling)	✓	✓	✓
The Hundred (Modified - Supine Table Top)	✓	✓	✓
The Roll Up	✓	✓	✓
Rolling Back	✓	✓	✓
The One Leg Stretch	✓	✓	✓
The Spine Stretch	✓	✓	✓
The Swan-Dive (Preparation)	✓	✓	✓
The Swan-Dive	✓	✓	✓
The One Leg Kick	✓	✓	✓
Swimming (Modified - Quadruped)	✓	✓	✓
The Seal	✓	✓	✓
Sit to Stand (transition)	✓	✓	✓

	Children	Children & Adolescents	Adolescents
	Ages 5 - 8	Ages 9 - 13	Ages 12 - 18
		Magic Window	
Chapter 8 - Pilates Exercises for the "Magic Window", Ages 9 – 13			
The Hundred (Modified - Straight Legs Down)		✓	✓
The Hundred		✓	✓
The One Leg Circle (Modified - Both Legs or Top Leg Bent)		✓	✓
The One Leg Circle		✓	✓
The Double Leg Stretch		✓	✓
Single Straight Leg Stretch		✓	✓
Criss-Cross (Modified - Feet Down)		✓	✓
Criss-Cross (Modified - Table Top)		✓	✓
The Neck Roll		✓	✓
The Double Kick		✓	✓
The Spine Twist		✓	✓
The Teaser (Modified – One Leg)		✓	✓
Swimming (Modified - Opposite Limbs on Mat)		✓	✓
Swimming		✓	✓

Chapter 9 - Pilates Exercises for Adolescents, Ages 12–18			
The Hundred			✓
Double Straight Leg Stretch			✓
Rocker with Open Legs			✓
Corkscrew (Modified -Torso on Mat)			✓
The Saw			✓
The Neck Pull			✓
The Side Kick			✓
Criss Cross			✓
The Teaser			✓
The Teaser (Progression: Moving the Torso)			✓

Chapter 6
Pre-Pilates Exercises

Introduction

Pre-Pilates exercises are the starting point for any student of Pilates. They are fundamental to the method and should be experienced and practiced before moving on to the exercises in the following chapters. The better these fundamentals are understood, the more beneficial the subsequent exercises will be. These fundamentals can be used in preparation for the exercises in the subsequent chapters, or as topics of study in themselves.

Exercises Included in this Chapter

When preparing for any Pilates-based exercise program it is important to identify and develop the following:

- Breathing awareness
- Pelvic awareness and alignment
- Cervical awareness and alignment
- Rib cage awareness and alignment
- Shoulder girdle awareness and alignment
- Spinal mobility and core stability

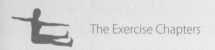

Breathing Awareness

In order to develop breathing awareness, it is helpful for the student to experience different types of breathing, such as:

- **Abdominal breathing:** the abdominal wall expands on inhalation and passively returns to the resting position on exhalation. This type of breathing promotes relaxation and might be used to calm students who are excited or nervous.
- **Rib Cage breathing:** the rib cage expands three dimensionally on inhalation and returns to the resting position on exhalation. This breathing also can be dynamic, in which case the ribs will move toward the center of the body with a forced exhalation. The inhalation can occur through the nose or mouth and forced exhalation occurs through the mouth.

If a structured breathing technique is not an option for the group, the most important consideration is that the students *just breathe* in whatever way is comfortable. To bring the body into balance, it is helpful to develop awareness of breathing patterns. Breathing is something that happens naturally, without thought. Bringing mindfulness to the breath, and breath to the exercise, can accomplish amazing things such as stress reduction, focus, spinal stability and mobility, and core control.

Can you breathe in through your nose? Can you do so for 5 counts, 10, 15? What happens to your ribcage and abdomen during the inhalation? Does the breath fill your bottom back ribcage and expand your side ribs? Or, does the breath stop moving somewhere in the top of your chest, throat, nostrils, or any other place?

Now, exhale through your nose. Can you do so for 5 counts, 10, 15? If not, imagine pursing your lips and blowing through a straw, or sighing, to slow the exhale. What happens to your ribs and abdomen during the exhale? Do you exhale for 1 count and have to inhale again? Does the breath stop moving somewhere in the process of the exhale? Do your abdominals push out or squeeze in?

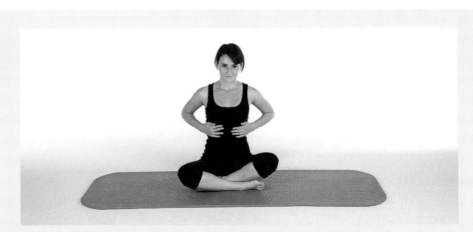

Now, put your hands on the sides of your ribcage.

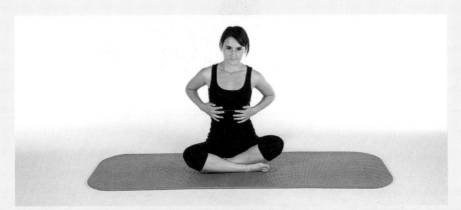

Can you inhale into and exhale out of your right ribcage?

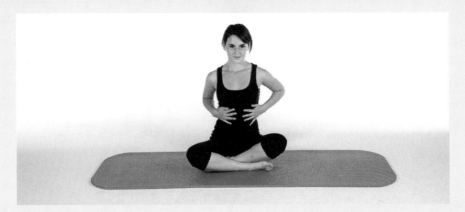

Can you do the same with your left?

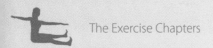

Pilates Breath

The Pilates breath is an inhalation and exhalation with control of the abdominal wall. Controlling the abdominal muscles during inhalation can facilitate movement of the rib cage, which can allow greater expansion of the lungs. With forced exhalation, more air is pushed out of the lungs. "To breathe correctly you must completely exhale and inhale, always trying very hard to 'squeeze' every atom of impure air from your lungs in much the same manner that you would wring every drop of water from a wet cloth" (Pilates, 1945). Let's practice.

Supine Breathing

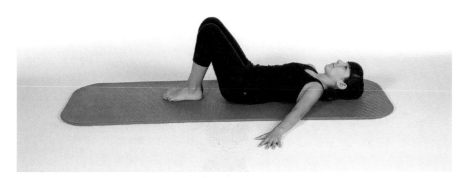

Lie supine (on your back), in the hook lying position (knees bent and feet on the floor), with hands by your sides, palms down. Notice if the area of your back from your shoulder blades to your waist is on or off the mat.

Breathe in through the nose for a count of 5, and as you inhale, allow your body to melt into the mat; feel your bottom back ribs and mid-back move gently toward the mat. Gently exhale through the nose for 6 to 8 counts while deepening your connection to the mat, and imagining the spine getting wider and longer.

Do this exercise 5 times and notice the difference between the 1st and 5th time.

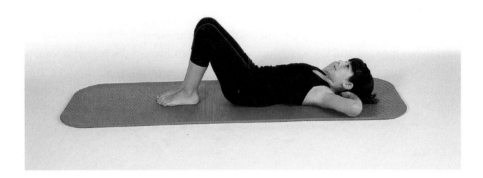

Now try the same exercise with the hands clasped behind the head.

Notice, if you open your elbows, do your ribs pop up off the mat? Be mindful not to force the arms open if the shoulders are tight. Work within your own range and focus on the rib cage relaxing into the mat. The arms will gradually open without force as the mid-back, chest, and shoulders relax.

Seated Breathing

You can practice the same breathing exercise while sitting on the mat in a cross-legged 'tailor' position. Place the hands on the bottom of the rib cage.

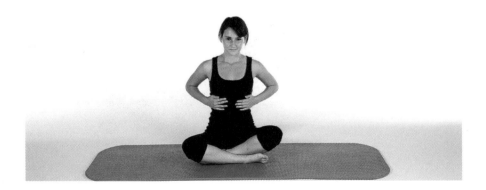

As you practice Pilates, you will be able to use the breath not only to move the rib cage but also to control and facilitate movements of the spine and limbs. While practicing, remember to be mindful of the breath in each and every exercise.

Pelvic Awareness and Alignment

To bring awareness to the alignment of the pelvis, lie supine in the hook lying position (knees bent and feet on the floor). Notice the curves of the spine. As you inhale and exhale begin to rock your pelvis forward and back (so the low back moves toward the mat and then lifts away from the mat) without moving the head, shoulders, chest, or gripping the feet. Then, allow the head, shoulders and ribs to move as the pelvis moves. Notice the changes in the curves of the spine.

Hook Lying

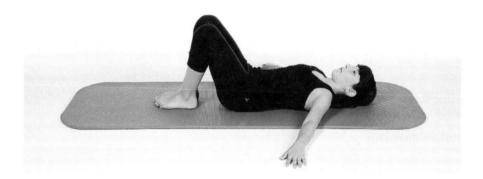

Posterior Pelvic Tilt

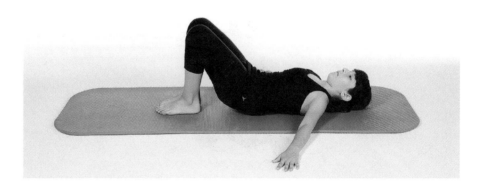

Anterior Pelvic Tilt

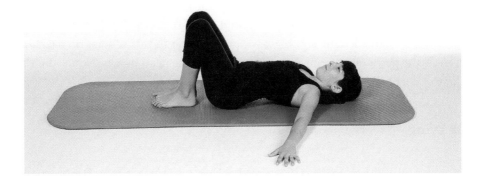

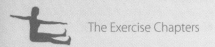

Cervical Awareness and Alignment

To bring awareness to the position of the head and neck, lie supine in the hook lying position (knees bent and feet on the floor). Inhale through the nose completely and upon exhalation, relax all of the tension in the neck, shoulders, and rib cage. Notice the curve of the neck. Begin to tilt the chin gently forward and back without moving the shoulders, rib cage, or pelvis. Then, allow the pelvis, shoulders and ribs to move as the head moves. Notice the change in the curve of the neck.

Hook Lying

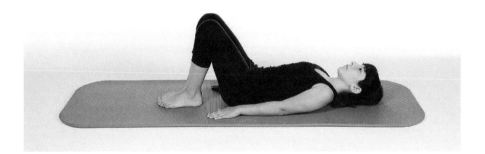

Cervical Extension

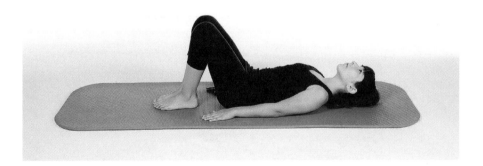

Cervical Flexion

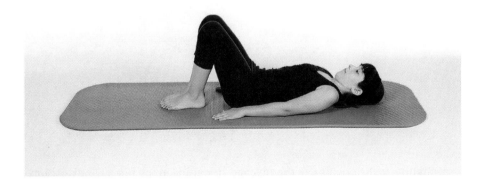

Imagery: Imagine drawing a straight line on the ceiling with your nose.

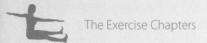

Rib Cage Awareness and Alignment

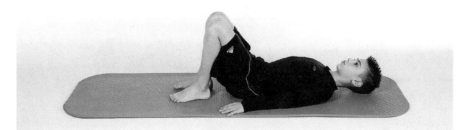

To bring awareness to the position of the rib cage, lie supine in the hook lying position (knees bent and feet on the floor), with arms lying along the sides of the body, palms down. Inhale through the nose completely and notice where your breath goes. Are you able to breathe into the back and sides of your lungs and feel the rib cage move? Exhale completely and notice if there are gaps between your spine and the mat after the rib cage relaxes.

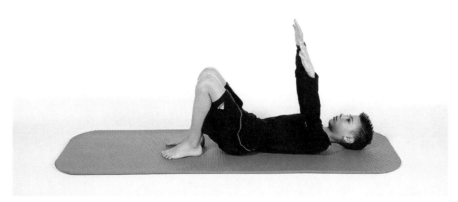

Raise the arms, shoulder width, straight up to the sky. Inhale and exhale, feeling the rib cage relax into the mat.

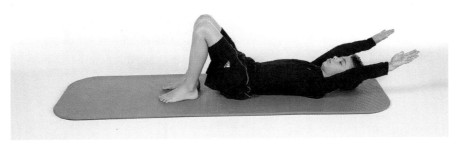

Inhale and exhale, and at the end of the exhale, move the arms backward, elbows straight, only as far as the ribs can stay connected to the floor. Inhale again (keeping arms back) and gently arch the upper back. Exhale completely (keeping arms back) and draw the rib cage deeper down, noticing more of the back of the body connecting to the mat.

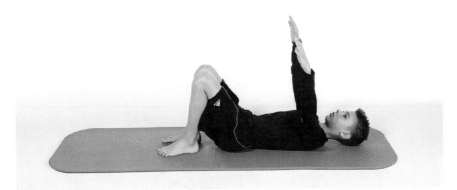

Raise the arms, shoulder width, straight up to the sky. Inhale and exhale completely feeling the rib cage relax. Notice what happens to the torso.

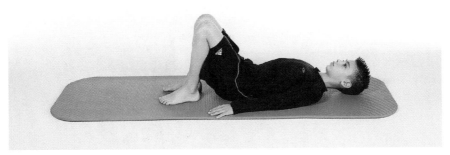

Exhale completely and feel the difference in the rib cage placement in the body.

Arm Scissors

Arm Scissors supine can provide a different challenge to your ability to keep your torso in a neutral position. Notice when scissoring the arms if the body rotates or moves differently than when you move the arms together. When moving arms overhead, allow arms back only as far as the shoulders and rib cage will allow before losing the connection between the two.

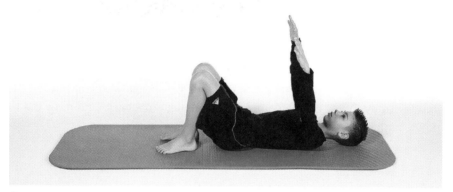

Raise the arms, shoulder width, straight up to the sky. Inhale and exhale completely feeling the rib cage relax.

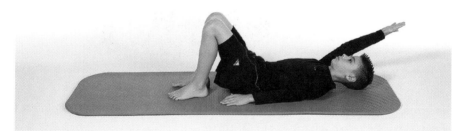

Inhale and exhale, and at the end of the exhale, keeping the rib cage still, reach the right arm back and the left arm down.

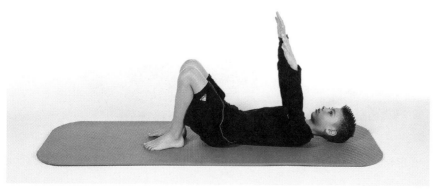

Inhale to return the arms to the sky. Exhale again in place, allowing the rib cage to relax.

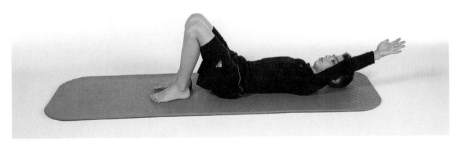

Inhale and exhale, and at the end of the exhale, keeping the rib cage still, reach the left arm back and the right arm down.

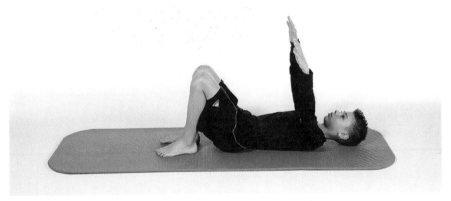

Inhale to return the arms up to the sky.

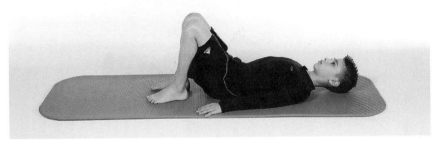

Exhale and bring the arms back down to the mat to rest completely.

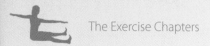

Shoulder Girdle Awareness and Alignment

Shoulder girdle awareness can be taught in supine, prone, sitting, or standing.

Supine

Shrugging up

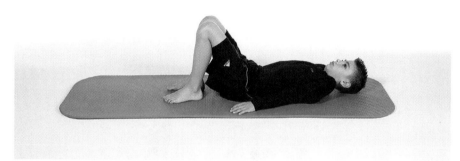

Lie supine (on your back), in the hook lying position (knees bent and feet on the floor), with hands by your sides, palms down. Inhale completely, shrugging the shoulders straight up to the ears.

Gliding down

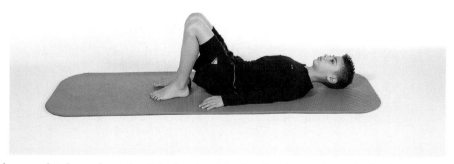

Exhale completely, and gently glide the shoulder blades down along the back and away from the ears.

Hugging the Moon

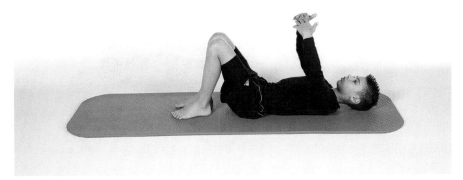

Raise the arms to the sky, backs of the shoulder blades connected to the mat. Inhale completely raising the shoulders off the floor, and reach hands up as if you were hugging the moon (this separates the shoulder blades on the back).

Opening Arms

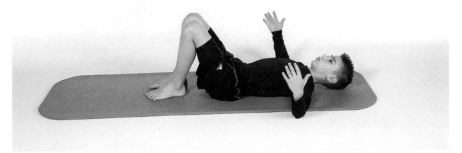

Exhale completely and draw the shoulder blades toward each other as the arms open. The backs of the shoulder blades resume their connection to the mat.

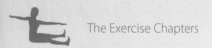

Prone

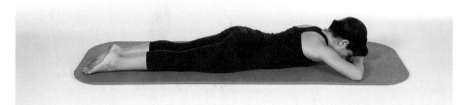

Lie prone (on your stomach), place the hands together under the forehead, elbows wide. Inhale completely, feeling the upper back expand across the width of the shoulders. Exhale completely and gently draw the shoulder blades down without losing the sense of width. Relax in position.

Shrugging up

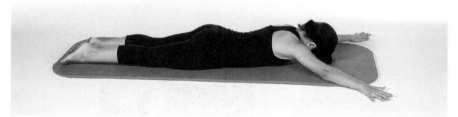

Reach arms forward along the floor, pressing palms down. Inhale completely shrugging shoulders up toward the ears.

Gliding down

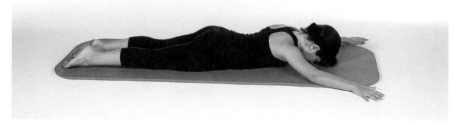

Exhale completely gently gliding the shoulder blades down.

Airplane Arms

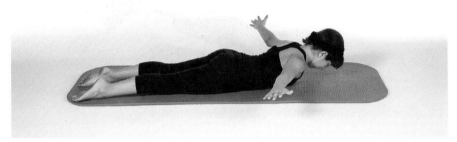

Reach arms out to sides (like an airplane), palms down and arms and upper body hovering above the floor. Inhale completely.

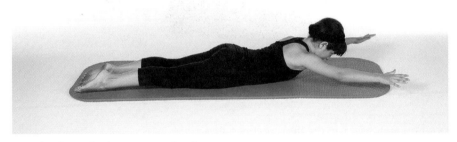

Exhale completely and raise arms up by the ears.

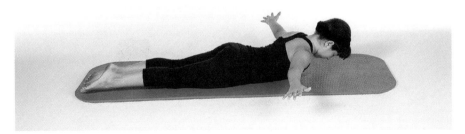

Inhale completely bringing arms back to sides.

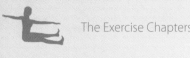
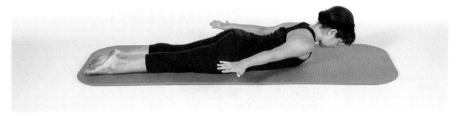

Exhale completely and bring arms down alongside the body.

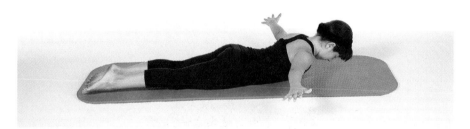

Inhale completely bringing arms back to sides.

Exhale completely and rest the body on the mat.

Reciprocal movement

The airplane exercise can be made more challenging by using reciprocal arm movements.

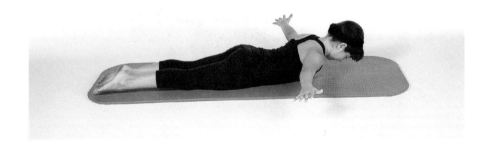

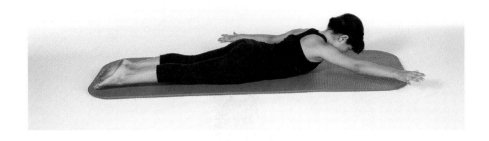

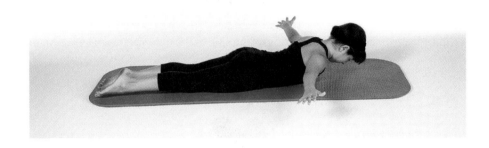

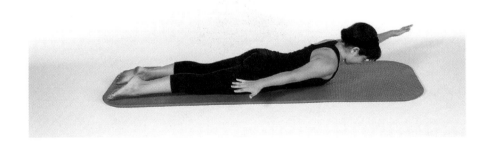

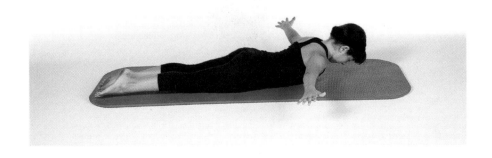

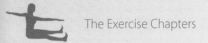

Sitting

Shrugging

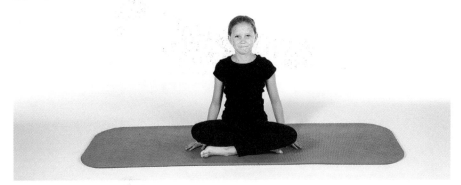

Sit in the cross-legged 'tailor' position, arms by the side of the body, palms of hands on the mat.

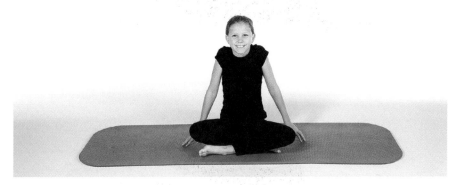

Inhale completely and shrug the shoulders up to the ears.

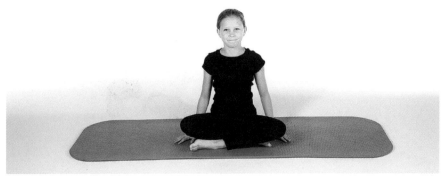

Exhale completely and return the shoulders down.

Hug a Tree

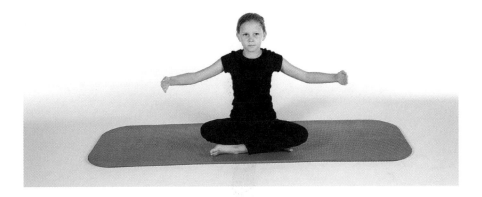

Sit in the cross-legged 'tailor' position, reach arms out to the sides, shoulders wide, keeping energy in the arms and fingertips.

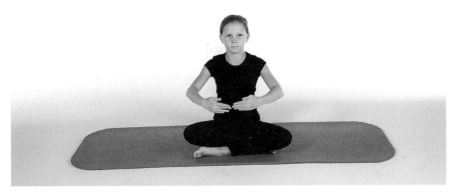

Inhale completely and "Hug a Tree" with the arms, as the back widens across the shoulder blades.

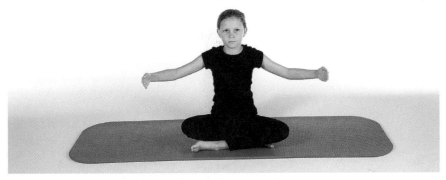

Return to starting position by exhaling completely, keeping energy in the arms and fingertips.

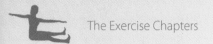

Standing

The "Shrugging" and "Hug a Tree" exercises above can also be done in the standing position.

Shrugging

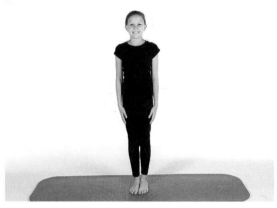

Stand with shoulders relaxed.

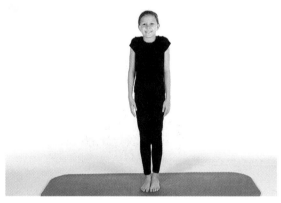

Inhale completely and shrug the shoulders straight up to the ears.

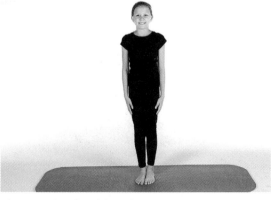

Exhale completely and return the shoulders down.

Hug a Tree

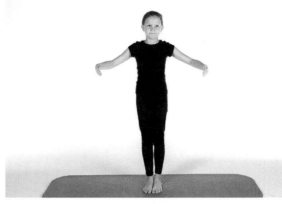

In standing, reach arms out to the sides, shoulders wide, keeping energy in the arms and fingertips.

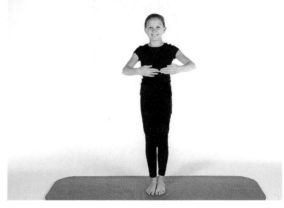

Inhale completely and "Hug a Tree" with the arms, as the back widens across the shoulder blades.

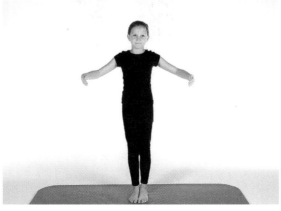

Return to starting position by exhaling completely, keeping energy in the arms and fingertips.

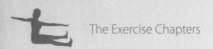

Spinal Mobility and Core Stability

Spine Mobility Exercises

Spinal mobilization should be considered in all planes of movement. Spinal mobilization exercises move the spine in 'flexion', 'extension', 'rotation', and 'side bending'. The full exercise program in Chapters 7 through 9 addresses *all* ranges of motion, whereas the following exercises are simply for the purpose of warm-up and awareness.

The Cat

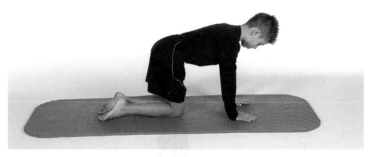

Kneel on all fours with knees lined up under the hips, and arms lined up under the shoulders. In this position, at the start and completion of the exercise, imagine the belly button holding a chain up off the floor, and the arms pushing the floor away.

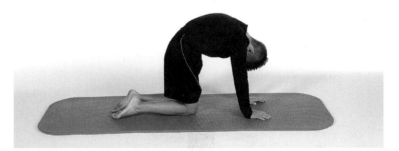

Inhale completely and round the back, curling both the tail and pelvis, and head and upper back, down and in. Continue to push the floor away and hold the imaginary chain up with the belly button.

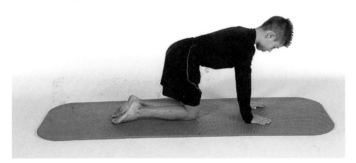

Exhale completely and return to the start position.

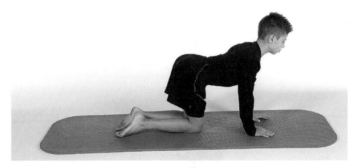

Inhale completely into a gentle upper thoracic extension. Imagine opening across the collarbones. Do not let the back sag. Reach the chest gently forward and upward and let the tail reach gently backward and upward.

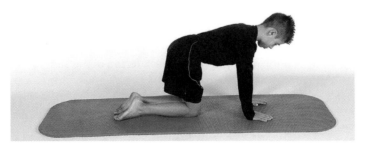

Exhale completely and return to the start position.

The Bridge

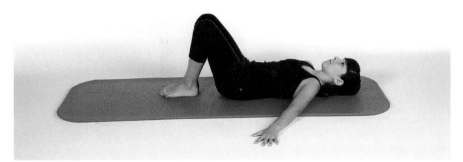

Lie supine in the hook lying position (knees bent and feet on the floor), with hands out to your sides, palms down, feet lined up with the sitting bones with equal weight in both feet, toes forward, and heels approximately 12 inches from the buttocks. Remember, in this position, to keep the chin gently drawn down and in (to lengthen the back of the neck), with the shoulders down and away from the ears. Inhale completely.

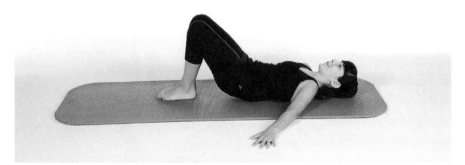

Exhale completely and begin to roll the pelvis and spine up in the air beginning at the tail bone and moving bone by bone until you reach the back top of the shoulder blades.

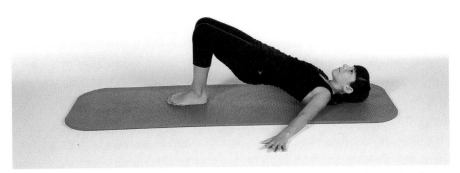

There is a diagonal line from the top of the knees through the body to the front of the shoulders. Inhale completely at the top of the position, and fill the lungs.

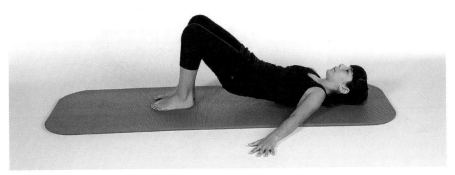

Exhale completely and roll back down from top to bottom, bone by bone . . .

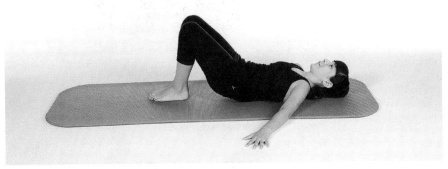

. . . until the pelvis is the last part to land.

While moving in and out of The Bridge, remember to push the floor away with the feet. When the pelvis lifts, imagine that the thighs and the knees will continue reaching over the toes.

Core Stability Exercises

Core stability should be considered in all exercises in all planes of movement. The goal is to attain and maintain the ideal alignment for each individual movement. The full exercise program and method was developed by Joseph Pilates to address stability of the body while moving the limbs, and will follow in this manual. For the purpose of warm-up and awareness we will initiate core stabilization, and focus on working in the supine position.

Hover

Lie supine in the hook lying position, arms behind the head, hands clasped together. Inhale completely and raise the upper body off the floor without bending or curling. Simply hover – spine straight, eyes to sky (head not tipped back), shoulders and upper back barely off the mat. Exhale completely and return to the mat.

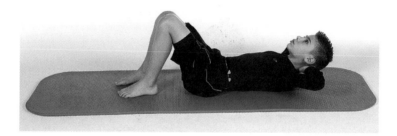

Rib Curl

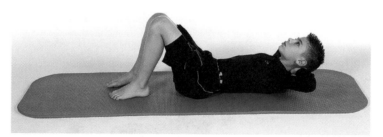

Inhale completely and initiate a "hover".

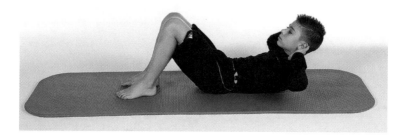

Exhale completely and gently curl the body from the rib cage. Remember to avoid gripping the hip muscles or feet or tucking the pelvis while curling the upper body. Inhale completely in the curled position, and then exhale completely to return to the mat.

Hip Folds

Lie supine in the hook lying position, arms to sides, palms down, feet lined up with the sitting bones with equal weight in both feet, toes pointed forward, and heels approximately 12 inches from the buttocks. Remember in this position to keep the chin gently drawn down and in, and the shoulders down and away from the ears.

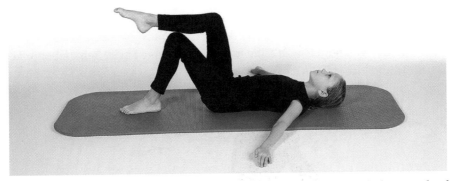

Inhale completely and raise the right knee to a 90-degree angle. Exhale completely and return to the floor.

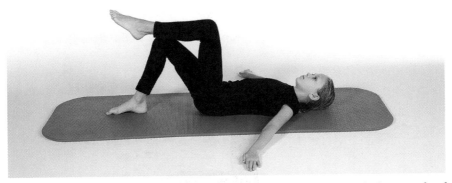

Inhale completely and raise the left knee to a 90-degree angle. Exhale completely and return to the floor. Be mindful to not change the position of the torso while raising and lowering the leg.

Toe Taps

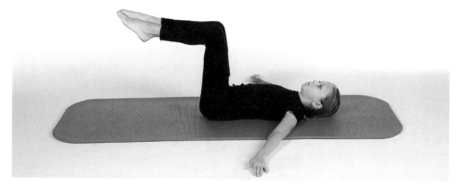

This exercise begins with both legs in table top, at a 90-degree angle. Remember to keep the chin, ribs, arms, and hips still during the exercise.

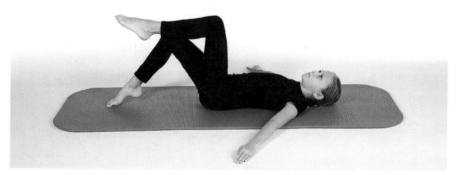

Inhale completely. Exhale completely and tap the right toe to the floor (left knee remains lifted and unmoving).

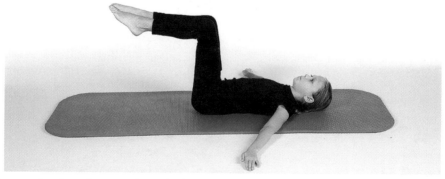

Inhale completely and return the right knee to the 90-degree position.

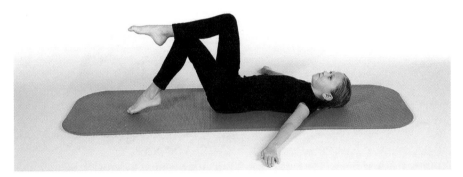

Exhale completely and tap the left toe to the floor. Inhale completely to return. Additional challenge can be created by initiating the toe tap on the inhalation and the return on the exhalation.

Double Knee Side Drop

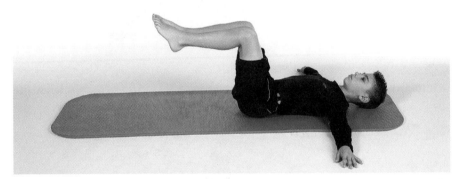

This exercise begins with both knees in table top at a 90-degree angle, with arms reaching out to the side, palms down on the floor. Remember to keep the chin, ribs, arms, and hips still during the exercise. Inhale completely.

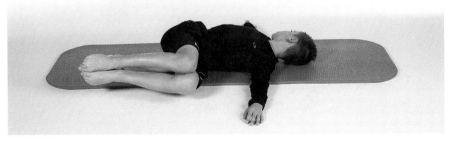

Exhale completely, gently dropping both legs to the left side. Inhale and feel the stretch in the torso.

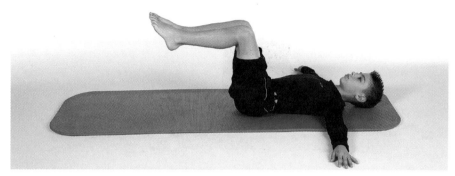

Exhale completely and return the legs to the 90-degree position by moving sequentially from the ribs, waist and hips. Inhale completely.

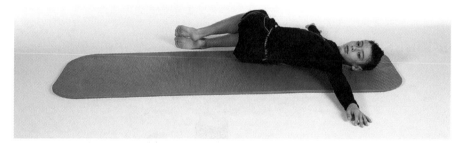

Exhale completely dropping both legs to the right side. Inhale and feel the stretch in the torso.

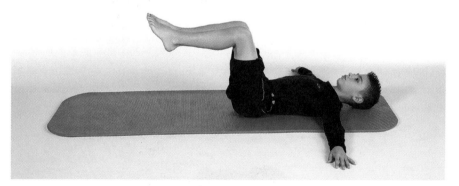

Exhale completely and return the legs to the 90-degree position by moving sequentially from the ribs, waist and hips.

Inhale completely and hold, then exhale and bring the feet to the floor.

Note

The experience can be varied by switching the breathing pattern.

General Modifications for Safe Positioning

- If the student's neck does not align properly on the mat, (if the chin is jutting toward the ceiling and the neck is extended) during or after the Pre-Pilates warm-up, it is advisable to use a small pillow to prop up the head and create length in the back of the neck.
- If the student is in a sitting posture and cannot sit upright without compressing the spine due to tight back or hamstring muscles, it will be helpful for them to sit on a rolled mat or small block.

References

Solomon, J., O'Brien, J., 2011. *Pediatric Skills for Occupational Therapy Assistants*, 3rd ed. St Louis: Mosby

Chapter 7
Pilates Exercises for Early Childhood, Ages 5–8

Introduction

As mentioned in Chapter 1, few Pilates exercises are appropriate for early childhood; however, appropriate selections for children ages 5 to 8 are included in this chapter. Teaching this group requires playful creativity, and cannot be based on learning by rote. Creative, natural variations of movement can be combined with selected Pilates exercises to create classes for this age group. Ideally, teachers working with this age group should have training and credentials in early childhood education. The teacher should understand the Pilates principles and age-appropriate Pilates exercises and use that understanding in the context of exercise as play and movement, rather than adhering to a strict exercise regime.

Exercises Included in this Chapter

- Imaginary Jump Rope Warm-up
- Standing Sequence
- Stand to Sit (Transition)
- The Hundred (Modified – Kneeling)
- The Hundred (Modified – Supine Table Top)
- The Roll Up
- Rolling Back

- The One Leg Stretch
- The Spine Stretch
- The Swan-Dive (Preparation)
- The Swan-Dive
- The One Leg Kick
- Swimming (Modified – Quadruped)
- The Seal
- Sit to Stand (Transition)

Note

Not all of the children pictured in this chapter are between 5–8 years of age. Also, Imaginary Jump Rope Warm-up and Standing Sequence are not traditional Pilates exercises, but have been included here as helpful preparation for the Pilates exercises that follow.

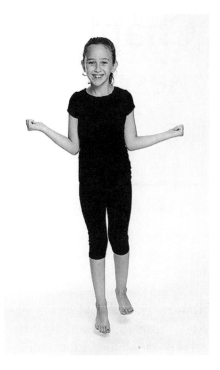

Imaginary Jump Rope Warm-up

Hold an imaginary jump rope. Place your right leg forward and left leg back. Jump in place and count backwards from 10–1, moving your hands as if you're using a jump rope.

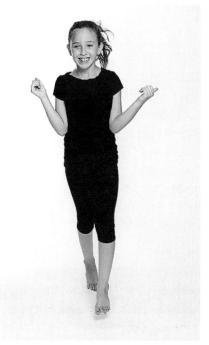

Switch to left leg forward, right leg back. Jump in place, counting backwards from 10–1, moving your hands as if you're using a jump rope.

Switch to the right leg in front, counting forward from 1–8. Then, switch to left leg in front, counting forward from 1-8.

Continue alternating the legs back and front while counting:
Backward 6–1,
Forward 1–4,
Backward 2–1,
And then switch legs for every count:
1, 1, 1, 1, 1, 1, 1, 1.

Standing Sequence

Boosting into Outer Space

Stand with feet together. Press arms firmly against
the sides of the legs.

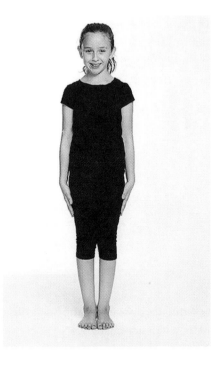

> **Imagery:** Press your arms against the sides
> of your legs as if you're a rocket ship ready to
> blast off!

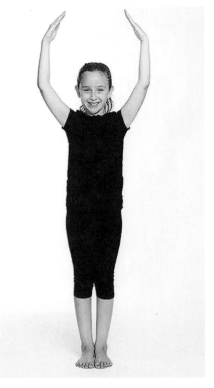

Inhale and raise both arms to the sky as if hugging
the moon. (The teacher can ask the children if they
want to hug the moon or the sun, and have the
children vote on which they prefer.)

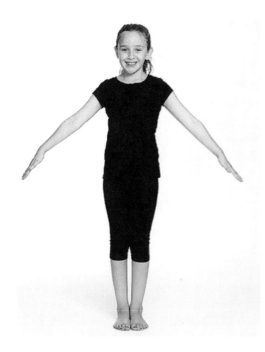

Exhale and return the arms to the sides. (The teacher can suggest that the children are boosting into outer space, and ask the children to say "Booost!" as they lower their arms.)

Note

Repeat the sequence above with the heels off the ground for a balance challenge.

Arm Stretch

Stretch right arm towards the ceiling.

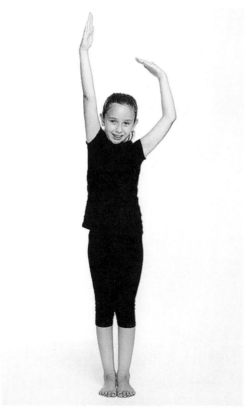

Stretch left arm towards the ceiling.

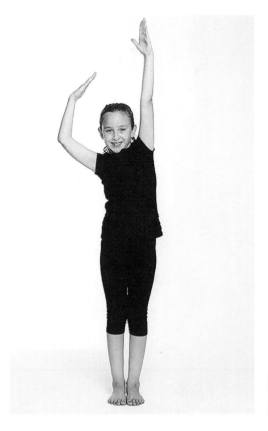

Imagery: Reach for the stars!

Note
Perform the sequence above with the heels off the ground for a balance challenge.

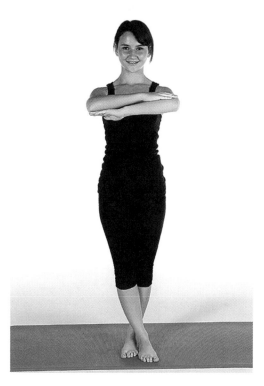

Stand to Sit (Transition)

Cross the arms, one forearm on top of the other, like a "genie". One leg is behind the other.

Gently and with control, lower yourself to the floor and sit on the mat.

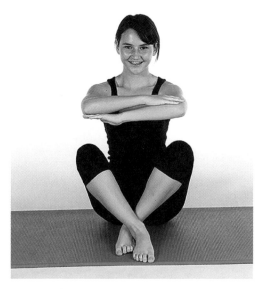

Note

This movement can be performed once as a transition between standing and sitting, or it can be repeated a few times for challenge and fun, ending in sitting.

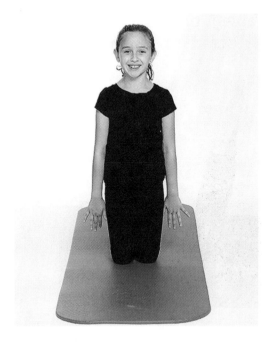

The Hundred
(Modified - Kneeling)

Kneel on the mat keeping the body tall.
Gently lift the belly and relax the tailbone.
Keep the arms by the sides of the body.
Palms face back.

Inhale slowly through the nose while pumping the arms for 5 counts. Then exhale slowly through the nose or mouth while pumping the arms for 5 counts. Perform 10 repetitions.

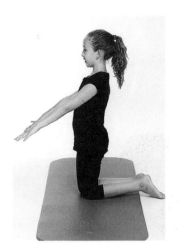
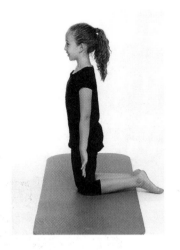
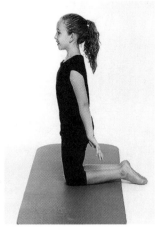

Note
Concentrate on keeping the torso stable while pumping the arms.

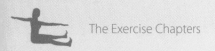

The Hundred (Modified – Supine Table Top)

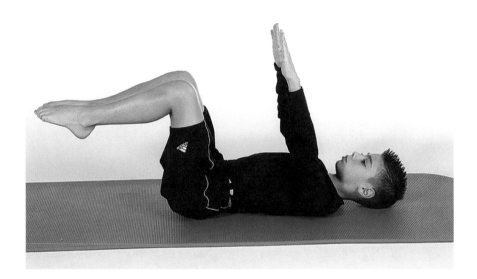

Lie supine with legs pressed together, in table top position. Raise arms to the ceiling.

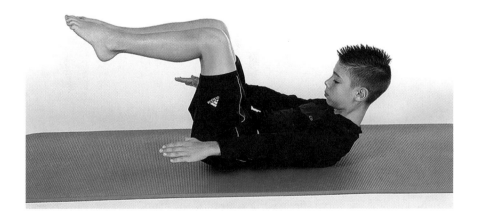

Keeping the back of the neck long, raise upper body and lower arms to hip height.

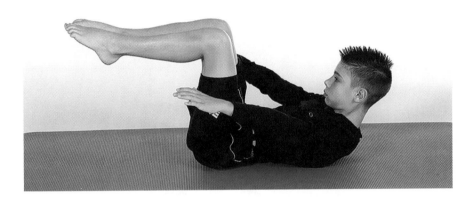

Inhale slowly through the nose while pumping the arms for 5 counts. Then exhale slowly through the nose or mouth while pumping the arms for 5 counts. Perform 10 repetitions. Keep the arms 6-8 inches above the floor.

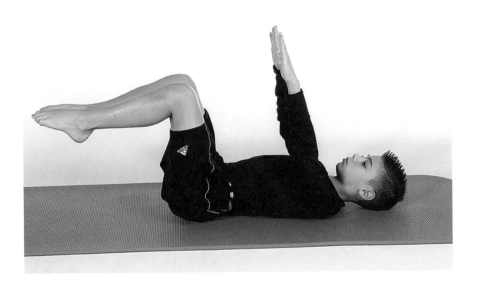

To finish, roll down with control.

The Roll Up

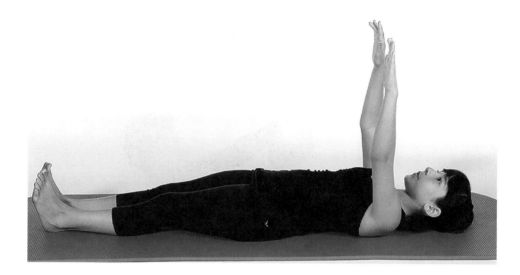

Lie supine. Reach legs long and together on the mat. Extend arms up to the sky making a "window" to look through.

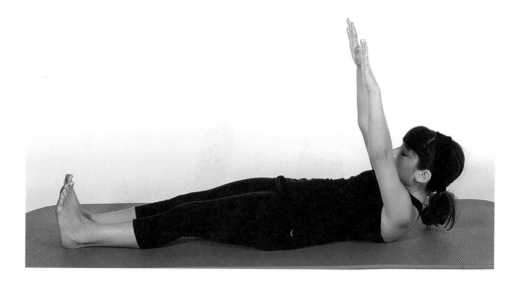

Inhale slowly; raise the head to look through the "window" of the arms. Keep the back of the neck long.

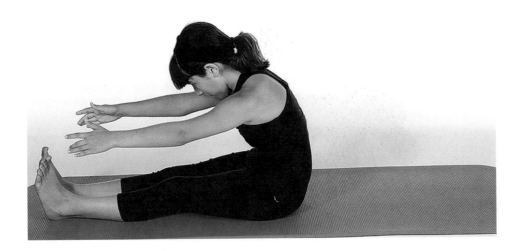

Exhale slowly; round the body upward and forward with the abdominal wall drawn in and up as the body stretches forward toward the feet.

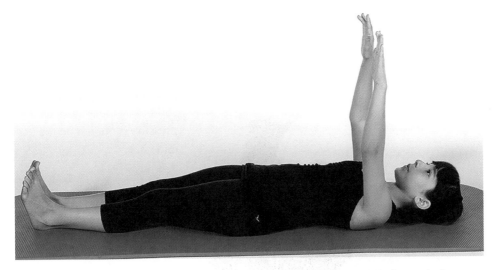

Inhale and slowly roll the body back to the start position with control, then exhale.

Perform 3–5 times. Finish in sitting position on the last repetition.

Imagery: The spine moves one vertebra at a time, like a string of beads.

Note
For an alternate arm position, try putting the palms flat on floor during the forward stretch.

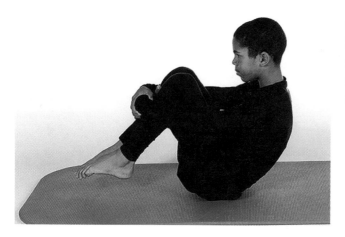

Rolling Back

Start seated, balancing on the back of the sit bones with the feet off the floor. Bring knees toward the chest. Hold the front of the shins.

Modification
Hands can be crossed over each other as shown; or the right hand can hold the right shin, and the left hand can hold the left shin. Alternatively, students can hold the backs of their thighs.

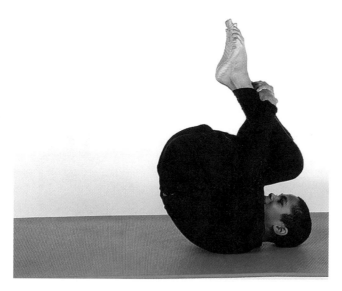

Inhale slowly, and roll back keeping the body in a ball shape. Roll onto the upper shoulders. Make sure that pressure is not put on the head and neck.

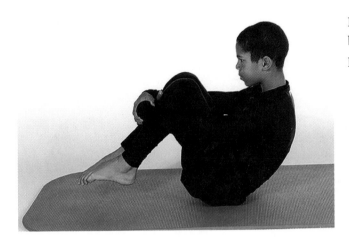

Exhale slowly and roll forward, back to the balancing starting position.

Complete 6 times.

Modification
To practice control, try holding the balance position without rolling.

Modification
Hold a ball between the chest and legs to keep the spine in a rounded shape. Avoid extraneous leg movement.

Note
Try to keep the feet off the mat during the entire exercise.

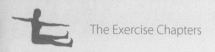

The One Leg Stretch

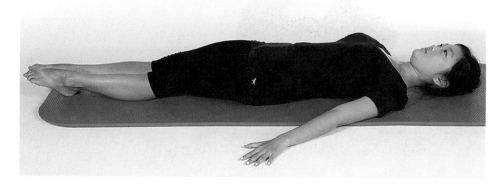

Lie supine. Keep arms long by the sides of the body. Keep legs together with pointed feet.

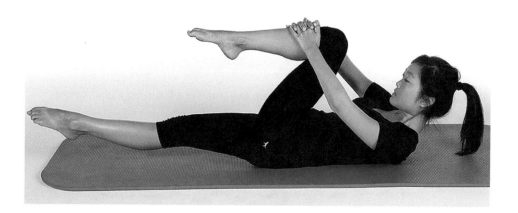

Bend the right knee into the chest with both hands clasped around the right shin. Keep the left leg straight and extended forward 2 inches off the floor. Raise the head off the floor, keeping the back of the neck long, eyes looking at the toes of the extended leg.
Inhale slowly and pull the right knee into the body. Reach the left leg out with energy.

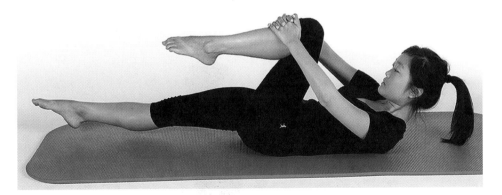

Exhale and switch the legs. Inhale slowly and pull the left knee into the body. Reach the right leg out with energy.

Perform the sequence above 5 times.

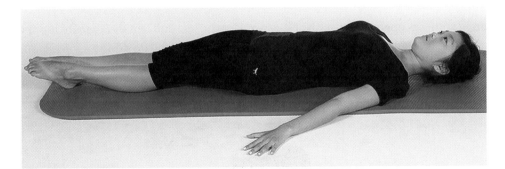

To finish, rest supine.

Modification
Instead of holding the leg by the shin, students may hold the leg behind the thigh.

Modification
The head may stay on the floor, or propped up with a pillow, ball, or a rolled towel.

Progression
Use alternating hand positions with right knee in, placing the right hand on shin near knee and left hand on shin near ankle. Reverse when pulling in the left knee.

Note
Keep the pelvis and low back stable while performing the leg movements.

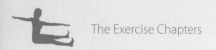

The Spine Stretch

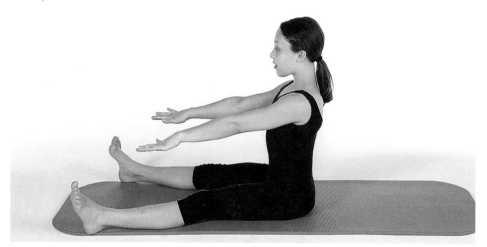

Sit upright with legs open to the width of the mat. Flex the feet and aim the knees to the sky. Do not allow the thighs to roll inward. Reach arms forward and inhale slowly.

Imagery: Imagine reaching the top of your head toward the ceiling while sitting on the floor with your back against a wall.

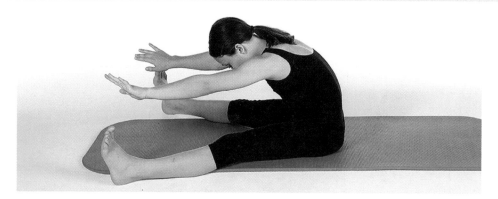

Exhale slowly and smoothly while curling from the top of the head down one vertebra at a time. Keep the pelvis stable. Keep the back of the neck long. Draw the abdominal wall inward and upward.

Imagery: Imagine resting your arms on an imaginary table.

Imagery: Imagine rounding your spine over a beach ball.

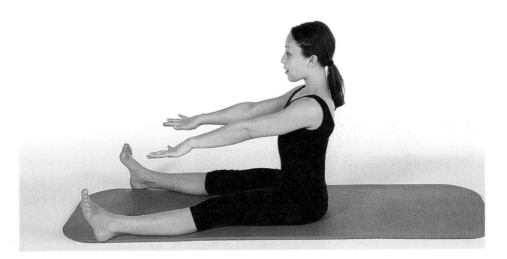

Inhale to curl up and return to the upright position.

Perform 3 times.

Modification
When curling forward (as in second photo), slide the hands forward on the floor between the legs (see example below). If hamstring and lumbar spine flexibility are limited, have the student sit on a rolled mat or blanket. Knees can also be slightly bent with feet flexed if hamstrings are tight.

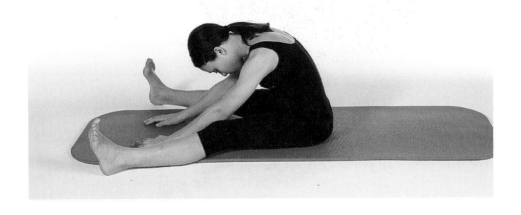

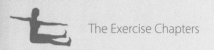

The Swan-Dive (Preparation)

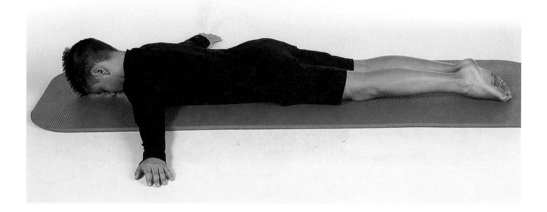

Lie prone. Reach arms out to the sides. Keep palms facing down.

Imagery: Imagine having "airplane arms", making the shape of a capital T.

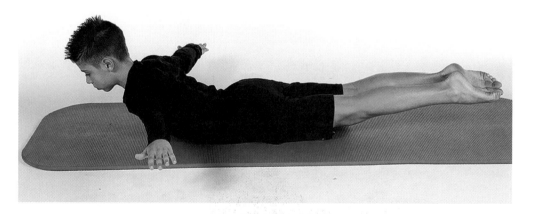

Inhale slowly. Lift the head and chest as high as possible keeping the lowest ribs on the mat. Keep legs together, and lift them off the mat with energy.

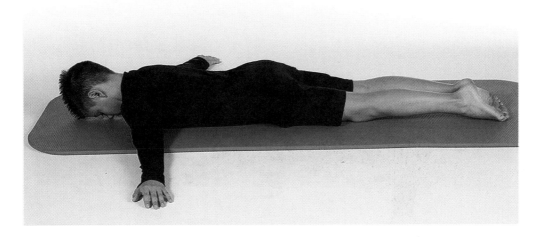

Exhale slowly and return to the mat.

Perform 3–5 times.

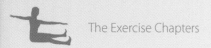

The Swan-Dive

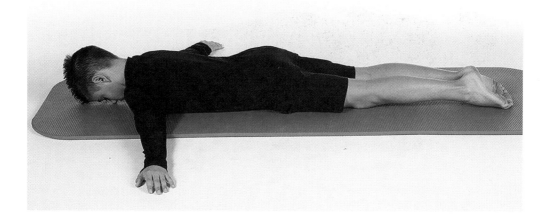

Lie prone. Reach arms out to the sides. Keep palms facing down.

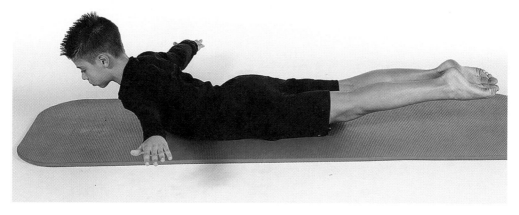

Inhale slowly. Lift the head and chest as high as possible keeping the lowest ribs on the mat. Keep legs together, and lift them off the mat with energy. Exhale and hold the position.

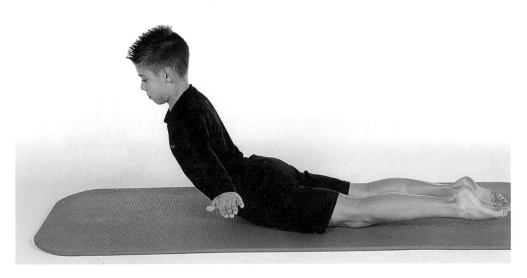

Inhale fully, rocking the body up.

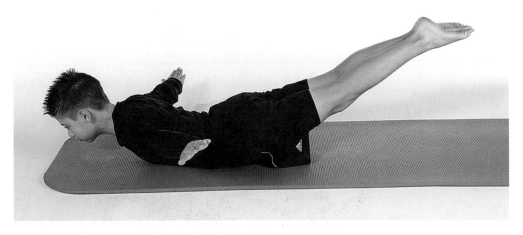

Exhale fully, rocking the body forward.

Perform 6 rocks.

The One Leg Kick

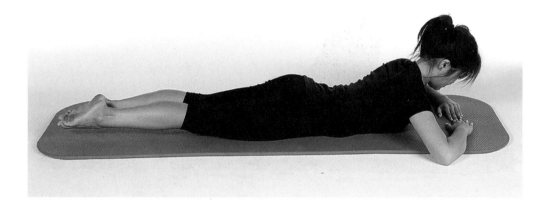

Lie prone. Place forearms and elbows on the mat slightly forward of the shoulders. Reach legs back and together 2 inches off the mat.

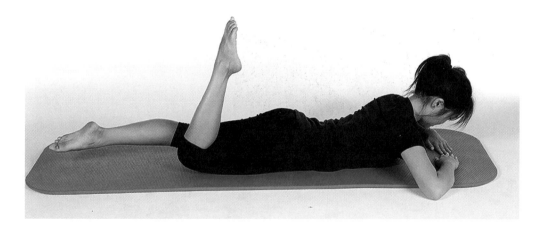

Inhale slowly, and snap-kick the right heel toward the buttocks. Exhale slowly and stretch right leg back.

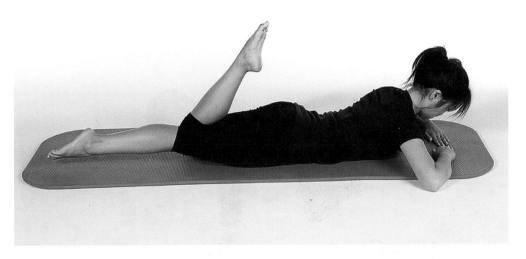

Inhale slowly, and snap-kick the left heel toward the buttocks. Exhale slowly and stretch left leg back.

Perform 6 times. Repeat starting with left leg.

Note
The torso should be in a gentle supported extension to ensure that there is no excess pressure on shoulders. Arms should be able to hover over the mat if requested. Both knees remain off the floor at all times.

Progression
For older children, flex the foot during the snap-kick to the buttocks. The foot points as it returns to the straight leg position.

Swimming (Modified – Quadruped)

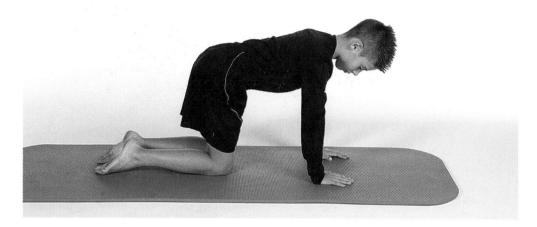

Kneel on all fours. Keep the arms aligned under the shoulders and the knees aligned under the hips.

Imagery: Think of the hips and shoulders being headlights facing down to the floor.

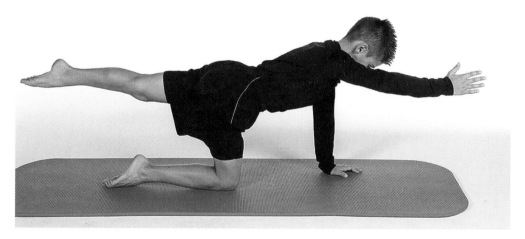

Inhale slowly and reach the right arm forward close to the ear without dropping the head. Reach the left leg backward without shifting the hips. Hold for 2 counts.

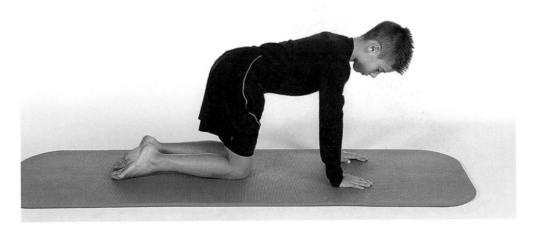

Exhale and to return to Quadruped.

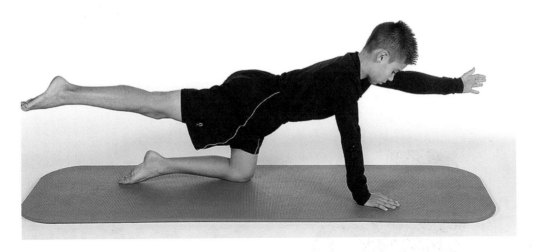

Inhale slowly and reach the left arm forward close to the ear without dropping the head. Reach the right leg backward without shifting the hips. Hold for 2 counts.

Perform 4–5 times alternating right and left sides.

Note
For this age group, the Quadruped modification is ideal for learning coordination and reciprocal movement with balance.

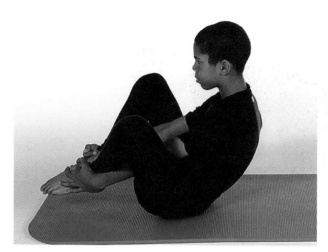

The Seal

Balance on the back of the sit bones with the arms "grapevined" under the calves, with hands wrapping around to hold the ankles. Keep the soles of the feet together. Keep knees slightly apart.

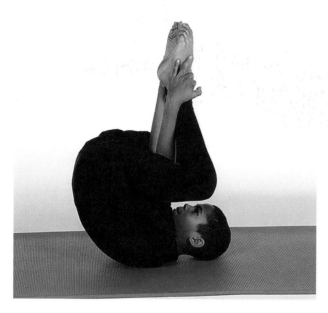

Inhale slowly to roll backward onto the upper shoulders. Make sure that pressure is not put on the head and neck. Clap the feet together 2 times.

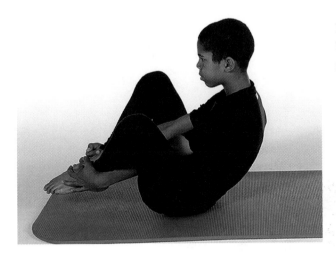

Exhale slowly to roll forward to balanced starting position. Clap soles of feet together 2 times.

Perform 6 times.

From the end balancing position, finish the exercise by crossing the legs and coming to standing position without putting the hands on the ground (see the Sit to Stand transition at the end of this chapter).

Note
Just for fun, bark like a seal when clapping the soles of the feet together!

Tip: Keep the back of the neck long in the curled position, with the abdominal muscles pulled in on both the backward and forward rolling motions.

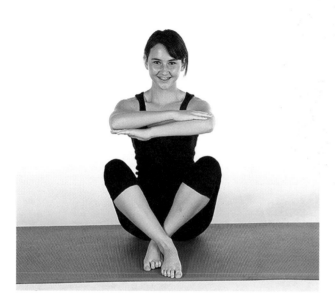

Sit to Stand

Cross the legs as shown and put arms into "genie" position.

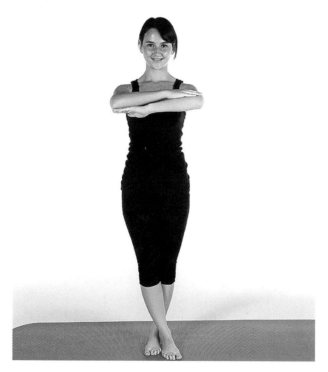

Push yourself up into a standing position. Then stand with legs together (uncrossed).

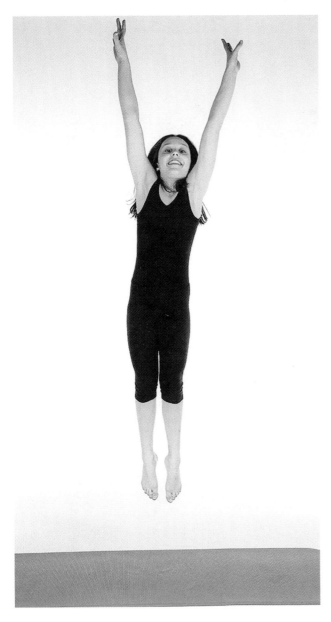

Once standing ...

JUMP FOR JOY!

Chapter 8
Pilates Exercises for the "Magic Window", Ages 9-13

(See Chapter 3 for more information on the Magic Window.)

Exercises Included in this Chapter

The exercises in this chapter build on the exercises programmed for Early Childhood students in Chapter 7.

- The Hundred (Modified – Straight Legs Down)
- The Hundred
- The One Leg Circle (Modified – Both Legs or Top Leg Bent)
- The One Leg Circle
- The Double Leg Stretch
- Single Straight Leg Stretch
- Criss-Cross (Modified – Feet Down)
- Criss-Cross (Modified – Table Top)
- The Neck Roll
- The Double Kick
- The Spine Twist
- The Teaser (Modified – One Leg)
- Swimming (Modified – Opposite Limbs on Mat)
- Swimming

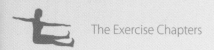

The Hundred (Modified – Straight Legs Down)

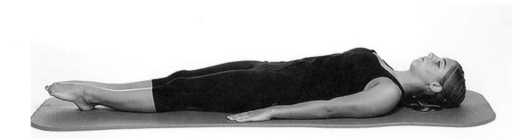

Lie supine with legs together on the mat, with the feet pointed.

Imagery: Imagine you are at attention like a soldier. For fun, children can vocalize "Hup!"

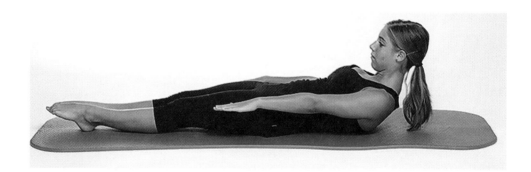

Lift the head, keeping the back of the neck long, with eyes gazing down at the toes. Raise the arms 6 -8 inches off the mat.

Imagery: Imagine your eyes are shooting darts toward your toes.

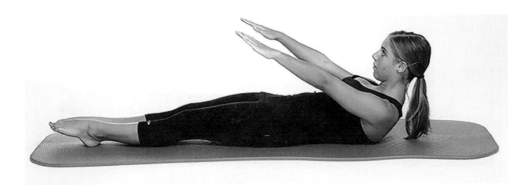

Inhale slowly through the nose while pumping the arms for 5 counts. Then exhale slowly through the nose or mouth while pumping the arms for 5 counts. Perform 10 repetitions. Do not let the arms hit the floor.

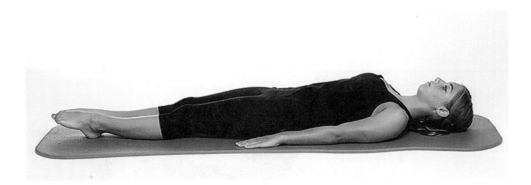

Return to the starting position and rest.

The Hundred

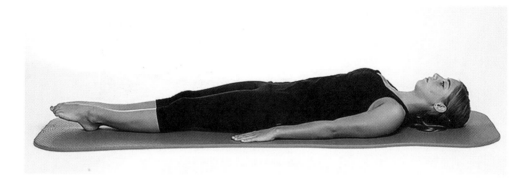

Lie supine with legs together on the mat, with the feet pointed.

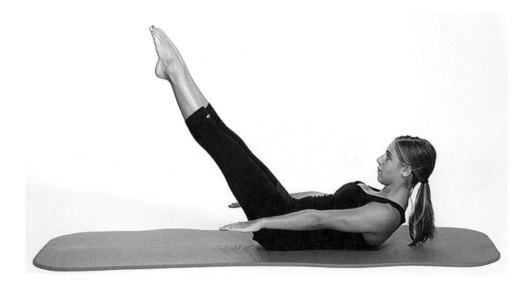

Bring the knees up to the chest, and then extend the legs out to 45 degrees. Curl up, lift the head and keep the back of the neck long.

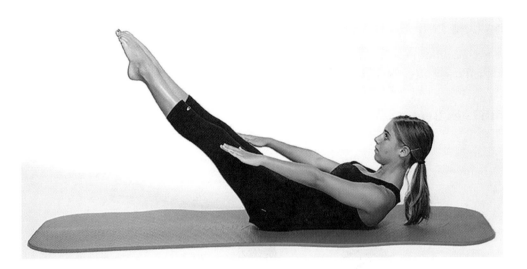

Inhale slowly through the nose while pumping the arms for 5 counts. Then exhale slowly through the nose or mouth while pumping the arms for 5 counts. Perform 10 repetitions. Do not let the arms hit the floor.

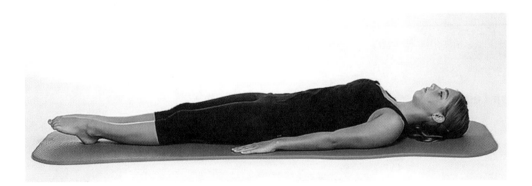

Uncurl with control, and return to the starting position to rest.

Progression
If the student can maintain their core stability and their torso's connection to the mat, they can try hovering their legs 2 inches off the floor.

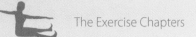

The One Leg Circle (Modified – Both Legs or Top Leg Bent)

The two modifications below may be used for younger ages in the Magic Window age group, and for those who cannot maintain core stability without strain.

Both Legs Bent

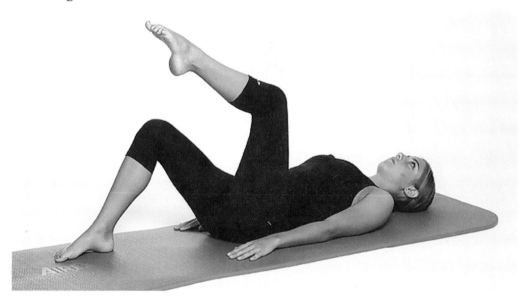

Top Leg Bent

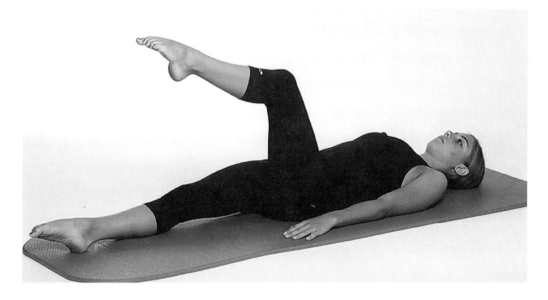

The One Leg Circle

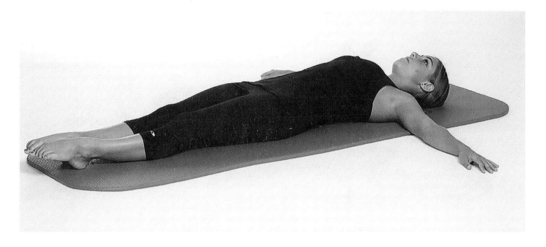

Lie supine with arms out to the sides, palms down. (Arms may also be placed by the sides, palms down.)

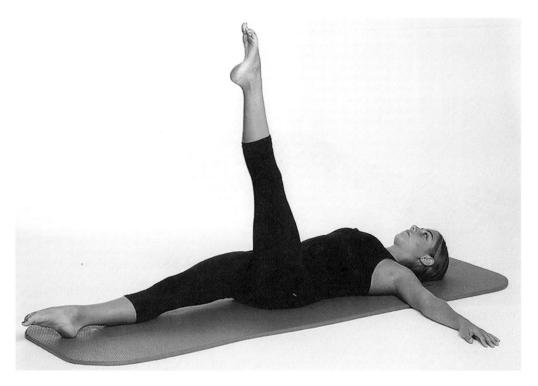

Bring left leg to upright extended position.

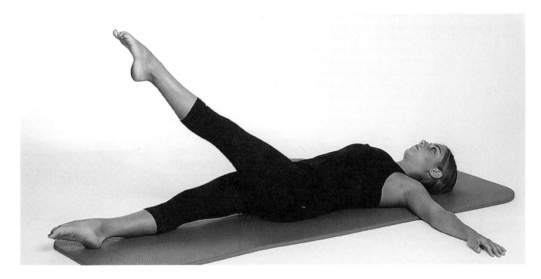

Exhale slowly *at the start of a downward motion* with the left leg while starting a right-to-left circle in the air over the right thigh.

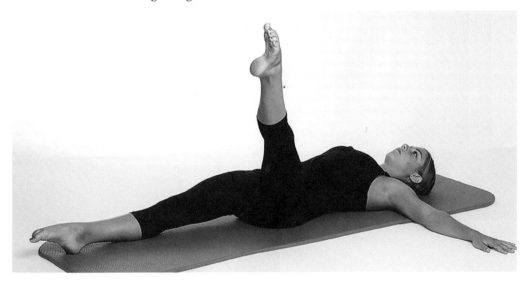

Begin inhaling slowly, *at the start of upward motion* with left leg completing this circle.

Perform 5 circles in one direction, and then 5 in the other direction. Repeat with the other leg.

Note Make leg circles only as large as the torso can be kept steady.

Progression
As a progression, the leg can fully cross the body allowing the pelvis to lift, making a big wide circle.

The Double Leg Stretch

Lie supine. Curl up, and keep the back of the neck lengthened. Bring the legs towards the chest, with feet and knees together. Hands are on the shins, with the elbows reaching out to the sides.

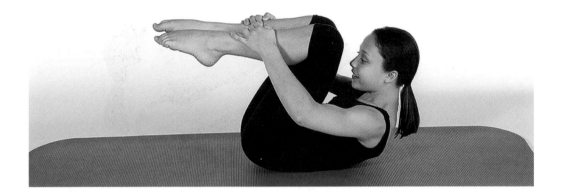

Imagery: Imagine you are holding a piece of paper between the knees.

Modification
The head can stay down on the floor, or can be propped up with a pillow, ball, or a rolled towel.

Modification
Students with knee problems can hold their legs behind the thighs, instead of on the shins.

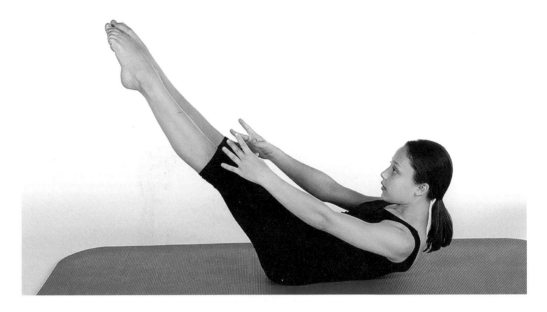

Inhale and extend the arms and legs simultaneously. Extend the legs out to a 45 degree angle, or lower, as long as the pelvis remains steady. Arms extend straight forward, or lower, directly by the sides at hip height.

Progression
For children at the older end of the Magic Window spectrum, arms can extend upward and backwards overhead alongside the ears.

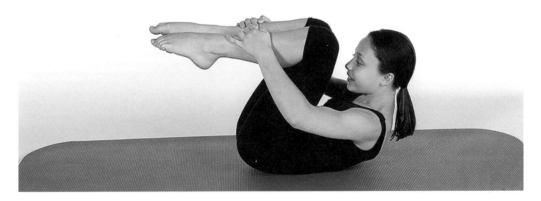

Exhale, and simultaneously return arms and legs to the starting position.

Perform this exercise 6–10 times.

Single Straight Leg Stretch

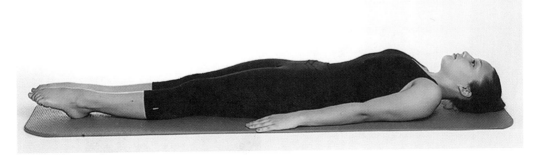

Lie supine. Keep the back of the neck long.

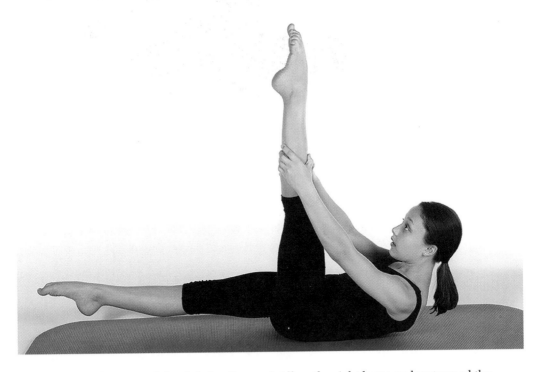

Extend the left leg up and the right leg forward. Allow the right leg to go low toward the floor, as long the position of the pelvis can be controlled. Reach the arms up with both hands on the calf of the upwardly extended leg, curling the upper body off of the mat. Inhale, and with the elbows moving out to the sides, pull the upwardly extended leg back toward the torso with a gentle double pulse.

Modification
The hands may be placed on the back of the thigh, instead of the calf.

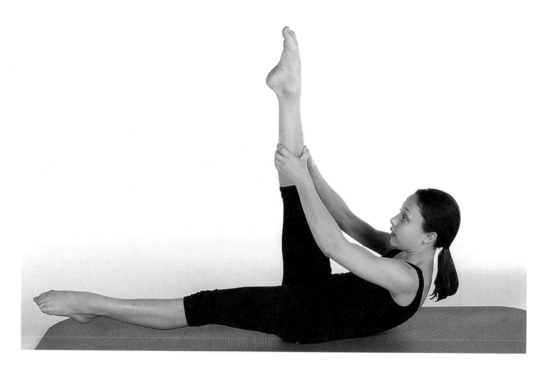

With a short exhale, "scissor" (switch) legs. Then inhale and pull the top leg back with a gentle double pulse.

Perform the exercise 6–10 times.

Imagery: Imagine there is a paintbrush attached to each of the feet.. As the legs "scissor", they paint two parallel lines in space that get darker and darker with each brushstroke.

Modification
The hands can be placed with fingers interlaced at the base of the neck, with elbows held wide and open, instead of on the leg.

Modification
As a modification, the head can stay down or can be propped up with a pillow, ball or a rolled towel.

Note
Maintain strong energy through the backs of the legs.
An alternate emphasis can be placed on the pulse of the lower leg reaching away.

Criss-Cross (Modified – Feet Down)

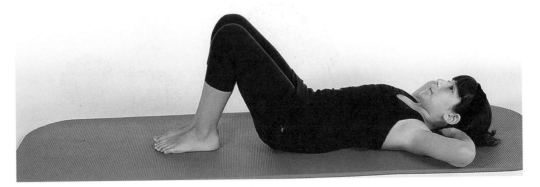

Lie supine, with knees bent and soles of feet on the mat. Keep the back of the neck long, Place the hands at the base of the neck, one hand on top of the other.

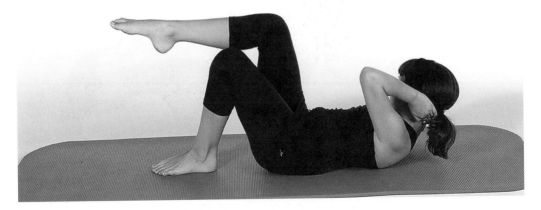

Inhale, twist and curl the upper body to the right, raising the right knee to the table top position.

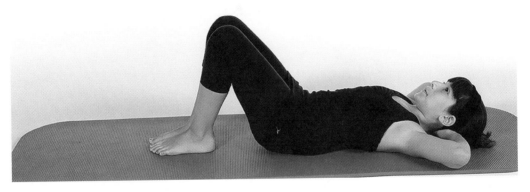

Exhale, return to the start position.

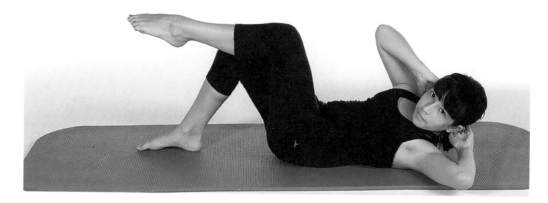

Inhale, twist and curl the upper body to the left, raising the left knee to the table top position.

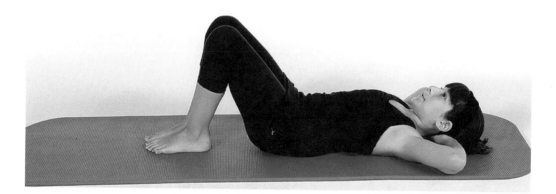

Exhale, return to the start position.

Perform the exercise 5 times, alternating between sides.

Criss-Cross (Modified – Table Top)

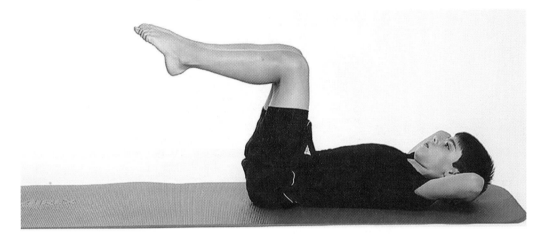

Lie supine. Keep the back of the neck long. Bend the legs in toward the chest to table top position, with knees and feet together. Place the hands behind the base of the head, one hand on top of the other.

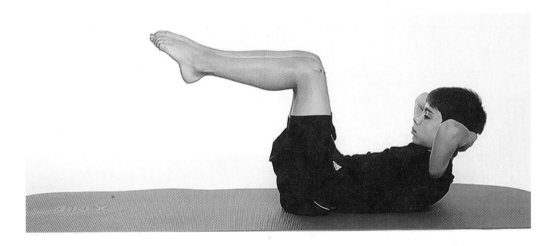

Inhale and lengthen through the back of the neck. Exhale to curl up, keeping the shoulder blades on the mat.

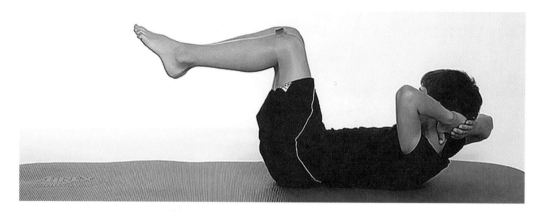

Inhale, and twist the upper body to the right.

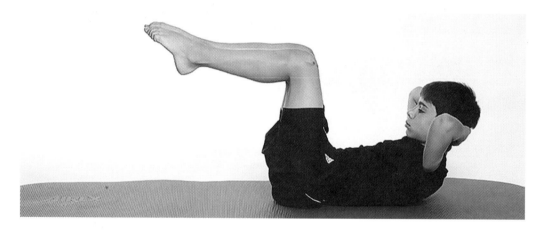

Exhale, and return to table top position.

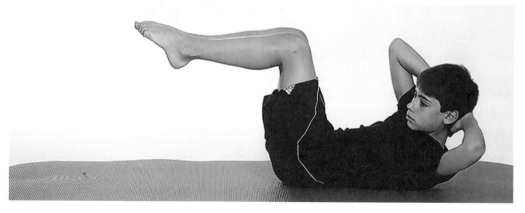

Inhale, and twist the upper body to the left.

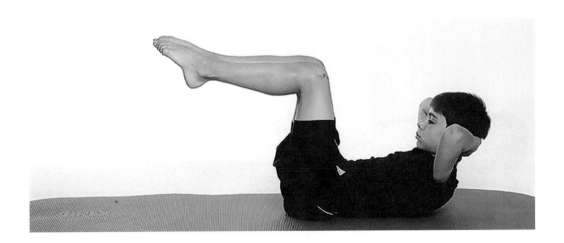

Exhale, and return to table top position.
Perform the exercise 5 times, alternating sides.

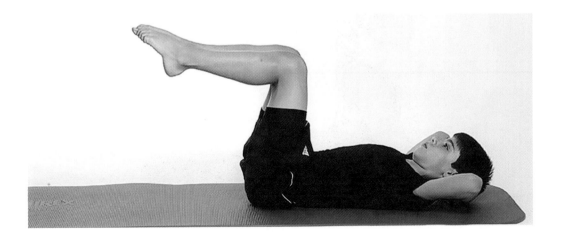

Return to supine, and rest.

Note
The lower body remains in table top position throughout exercise. Feel the weight of the tail on the mat.

The Neck Roll

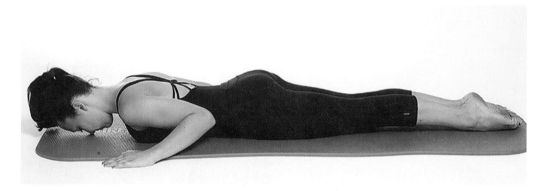

Lie prone. Extend the legs long and together. Place hands on the mat in line with the shoulders.

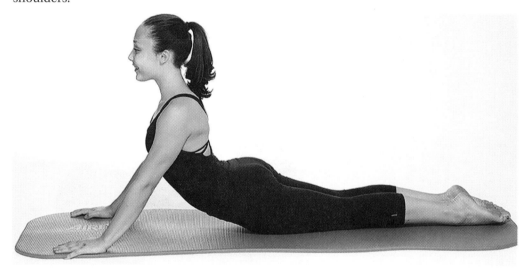

Inhale, and start extending the head and chest up off the mat. Exhale, continue the spine extension and extend the arms to a straight elbows. Relax the shoulders down away from the ears.

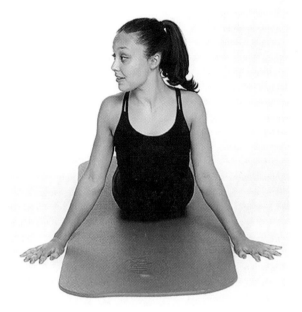

Inhale, turn the head gently to the right shoulder.

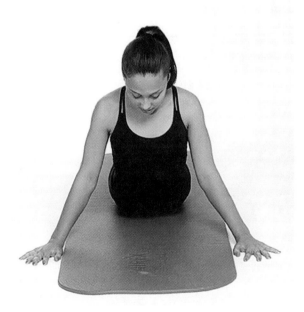

Continuing the inhale, lower the head and return to center.

Modification
Hands may be opened wider than shoulder width.

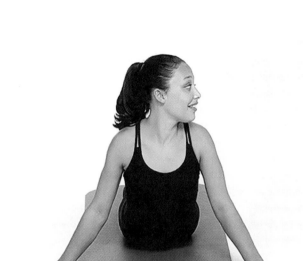

Exhale, and turn the head to the left shoulder, and then turn the head back to center with the gaze forward.

Repeat the sequence starting with the head turning to the left.

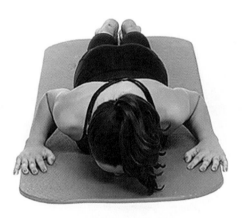

Inhale, bending the arms as the body begins to lower down toward the mat. Exhale, as the body continues to descend the rest of the way down to the mat.

Note
Support the lumbar spine by drawing the navel in and up.

Modification
Perform this exercise with the legs apart if there is excess tension on the lower back.

The Double Kick

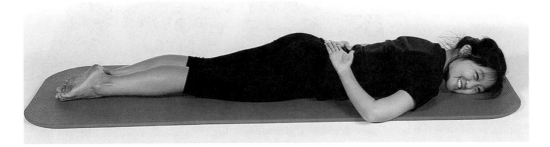

Lie prone. Turn the head to one side. Bring legs together and reach them long. Place the hands high up on the back, elbows bent to the side and pressing down. Place one hand on top of the other, with palms facing up.

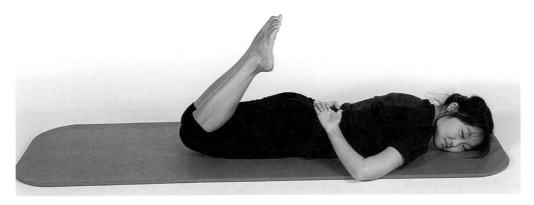

Inhale, then exhale keeping the legs together and snap-kick the legs towards the buttocks.

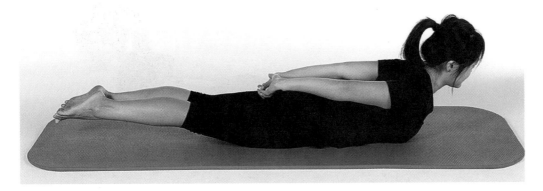

Inhale, and extend the legs out. Extend the breastbone up and away from the mat. Raise the arms from the body and stretch them back as far as possible.

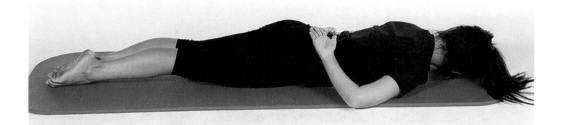

Exhale, and lower the body back down to the floor, placing the opposite side of the face on the mat.

Perform 3 sets alternating head position on the mat.

Note
Make sure the spine is in a long extension. Be careful not to compress the neck and lower back by lifting the abdomen, chest, neck and eyes so the front of the body supports the back of the body.

Variation
An optional head position is to rest the chin down on the floor, instead of turning the head side to side.

Modification
For younger ages, students can leave hands by the side of the body, palms facing down as shown below.

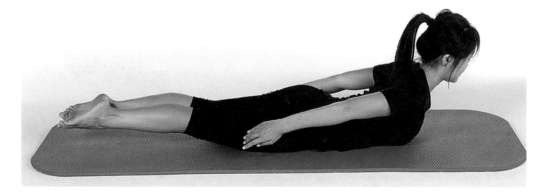

Simultaneously inhale, extend the legs, extend the breastbone up and away from the mat and rotate the arms so that the palms face the mat.

The Spine Twist

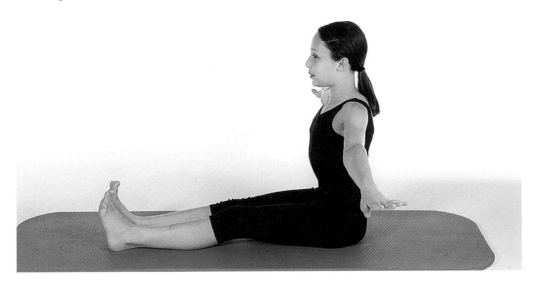

Start seated upright, with the legs extended long and parallel with feet flexed. Keep the head directly over shoulders and the shoulders directly over the hips. Open the arms to the sides, keeping them in peripheral vision, so that you can envision one line from index finger to index finger. Inhale to lengthen the spine, reach the head toward the sky, and reach the sit bones down.

Note
Make sure the rib cage does not flare forward.

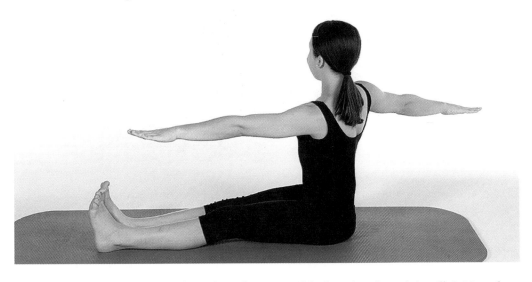

Exhale, and twist the spine to the right as far as possible, keeping the pelvis still. Initiate the twisting movement from the spine, not the arms.

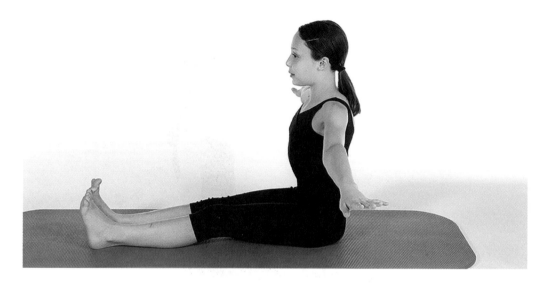

Inhale, the return the torso to the center.

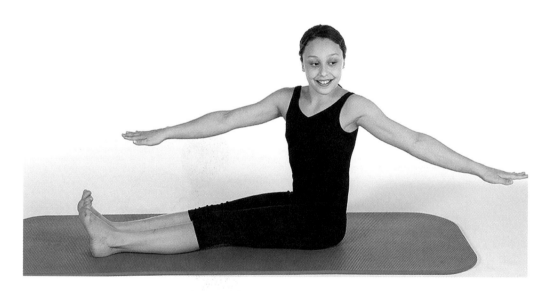

Exhale, and twist the spine to the left as far as possible, keeping the pelvis still.

Tip: Make sure the rib cage does not flare forward.

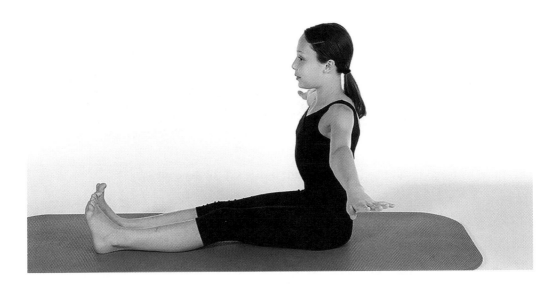

Inhale and return to center.

Perform 3 sets.

Imagery: Imagine the body to be a helicopter propeller as it twists.

Progression
Exhale, twist the spine to the right in a double beat. Inhale to return to the center.
Exhale, twist the spine to the left in a double beat. Inhale to return to the center.

Note
- The back arm leads the twisting movement, while the front arm stays in line with the collarbones.
- As the torso twists, the heels remain parallel to each other, as if they are against a wall.
- The arms can work in other positions, for example with elbows bent and the hands on the shoulders.
- Breathing can be alternated for a different emphasis, with the inhale on the twist and the exhale on the return.

Modification
The students can sit cross-legged, in "tailor" style.

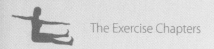
The Teaser (Modified – One Leg)

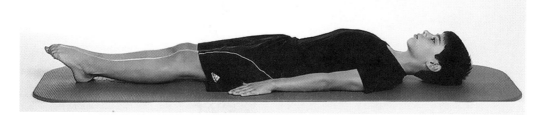

Lie supine with legs firmly together, with arms by the side of the body.

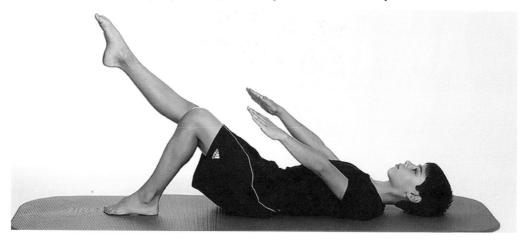

Bend the left knee, keeping the left foot firmly on the floor and extend the right leg, pressing the knees together. Reach the arms forward toward the extended the right leg.

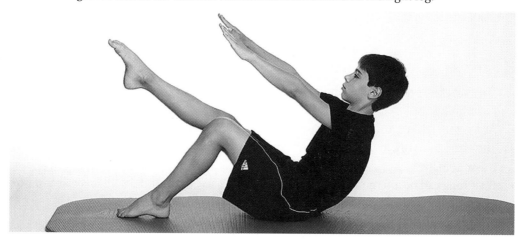

Inhale, and roll up into the modified teaser position onto the back of the sit bones with the abdominal wall drawn in and up.

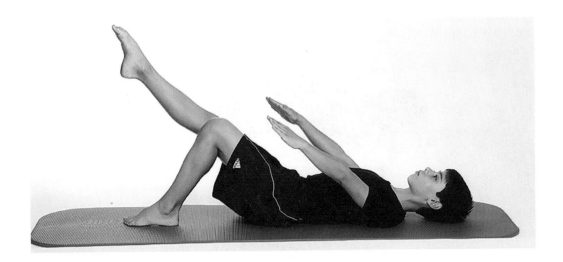

Exhale and roll down keeping extended leg steady.

Perform the exercise 3 – 5 times on one side; then repeat 3 – 5 times on the other side.

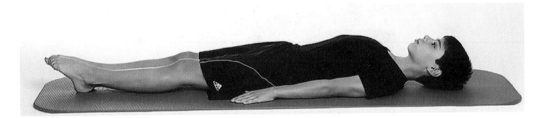

Finish in supine position.

Note
The roll up is initiated by inhaling into the back of the chest and ribs.

Caution: Avoid pulling the head forward in front of the shoulders while rolling up or down.

Swimming (Modified – Opposite Limbs on Mat)

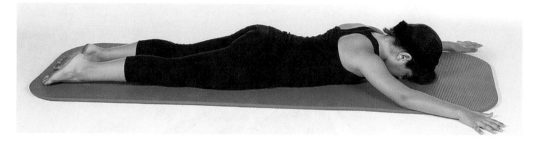

Lie prone with arms and legs extended on the mat.

Next, inhale, and raise the head and chest off the mat keeping hands and legs on the mat. Exhale, and hold the position.

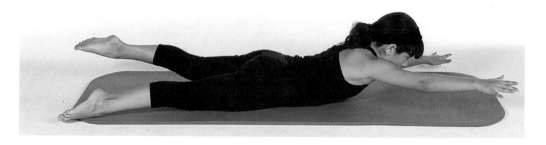

Inhale, and simultaneously raise right arm and left leg away from the mat. Keep opposite hand and leg on the mat.

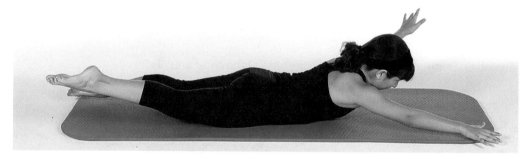

Inhale, simultaneously raise the left arm and right leg.
Exhale, return the limbs to the mat, keeping the head and chest off the mat.

Perform this sequence 3 to 5 times.

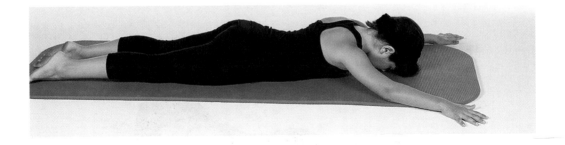

Return to prone position and rest.

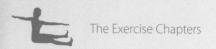

Swimming

To begin, inhale, and lift the head and chest off the mat while hands and legs remain down. Exhale and hold the position.

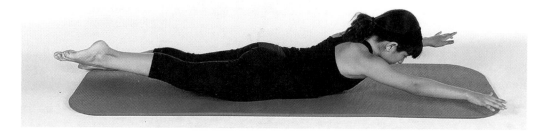

Begin to inhale and exhale in a natural rhythm while moving the arms and legs in a fluid and continuous swimming motion hovering off the mat.

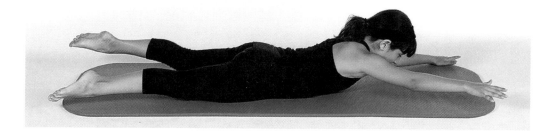

Continue swimming motion.

Perform the swimming motion while counting briskly to 10.

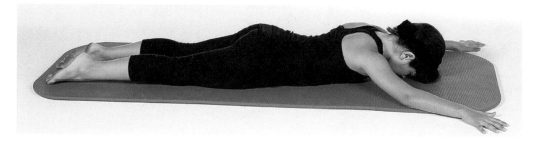

Exhale to prone position and rest.

Chapter 9
Pilates Exercises for Adolescents, Ages 12–18

Exercises Included in this Chapter

The exercises in this chapter build on the exercises programmed for the Magic Window students in Chapter 8.

- The Hundred
- Double Straight Leg Stretch
- Rocker with Open Legs
- The Cork-Screw (Modification: Torso on Mat)
- The Saw
- The Neck Pull
- The Side Kick
- Criss Cross
- The Teaser
- The Teaser (Progression: Moving the Torso)

The Hundred

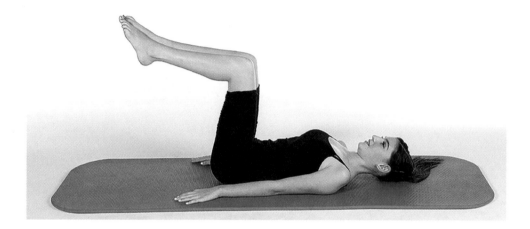

Lie supine and bring legs into table top position. Lengthen arms by sides of the body.

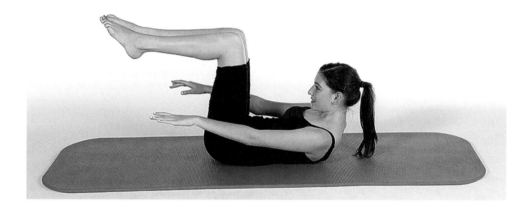

Inhale, nod head to look toward legs, and roll up to bottom of shoulder blades. Raise arms 6 inches above the floor and reach forward.

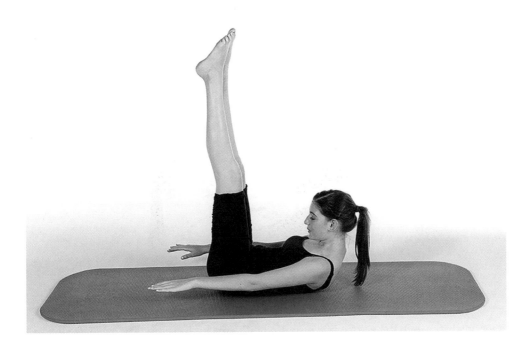

Exhale, extend legs toward ceiling.

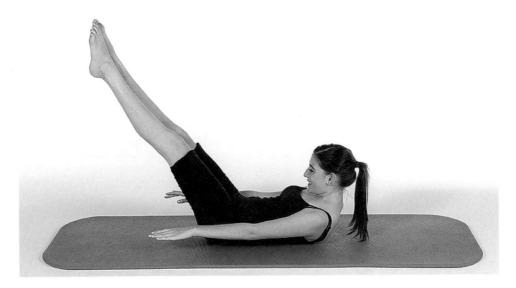

Lower legs toward floor as far as can be controlled without changing position of torso.

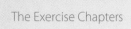

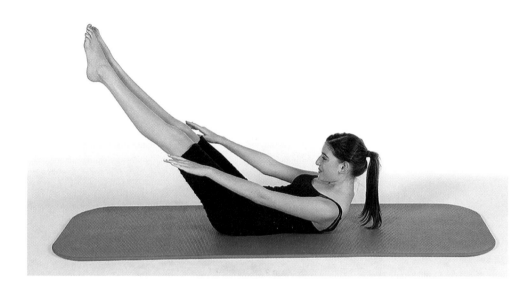

Inhale slowly through the nose while pumping the arms for 5 counts. Then exhale slowly through the nose or mouth while pumping the arms for 5 counts. Perform 10 repetitions. Keep the arms 6-8 inches above the floor.

Note
Concentrate on keeping the torso still and keeping the abdomen drawn in during the pumping arm movements.

Double Straight Leg Stretch

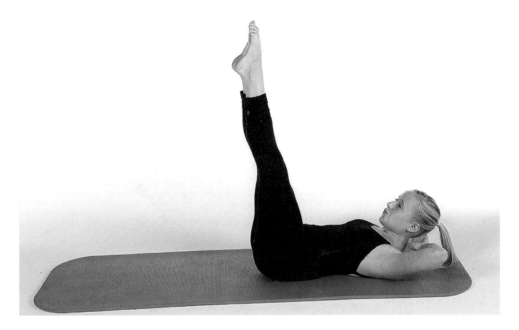

Lie supine with hands clasped behind the head and elbows wide. Bend the knees into the chest (the hip fold). Inhale and extend the legs straight up into the air. Exhale to raise the head and shoulders off the mat to the bottom of the shoulder blades.

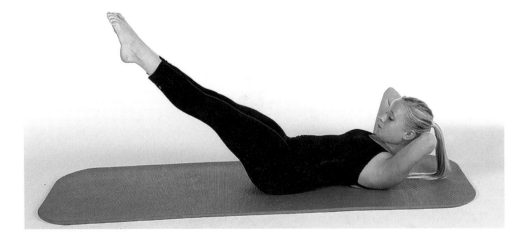

Inhale, extend and lower the legs (lengthen the front of the hips while maintaining abdominal control in order to not arch the back).

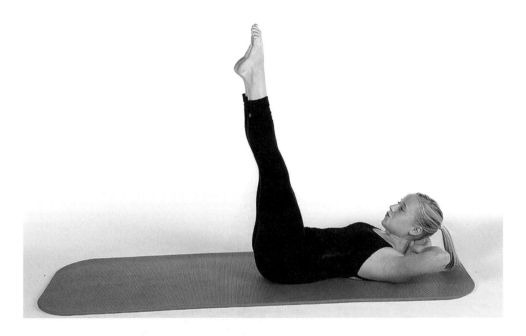

Exhale and return legs to reach to the ceiling.

Perform 6 to 10 times.

Modification

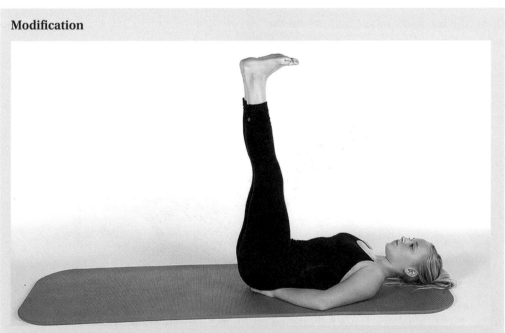

Place the hands under the hips, keeping the torso and head on the floor. The hands will help to keep the torso still while the legs are moving.

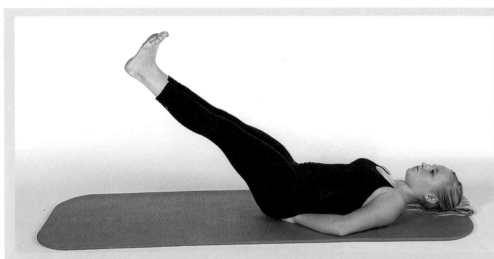

Inhale, extend and lower the legs (lengthen the front of the hips while maintaining abdominal control in order to not arch the back).

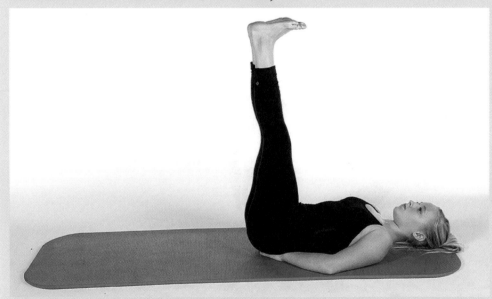

Exhale and return legs to reach to the ceiling.
Perform 6 to 10 times.

Rocker with Open Legs

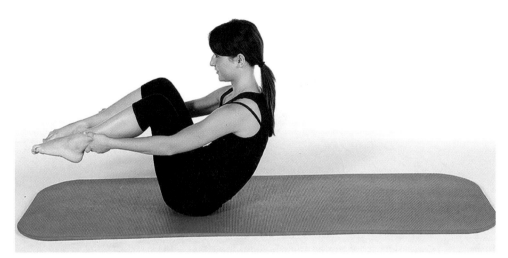

Sit toward the front of the mat, balancing on the back of the sit bones, with the knees bent in toward the chest. Hold the lower legs or ankles.

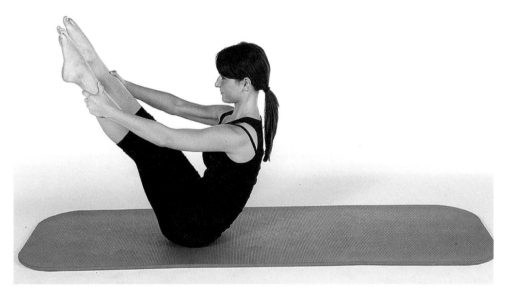

Inhale to extend the legs up and out, legs apart in a small "v" with arms extended. Flex the spine in an elongated curve while lifting at the waist and relaxing the shoulders.

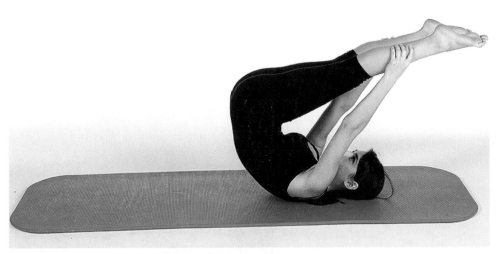

Exhale and roll the body backward, holding the legs throughout the movement. Roll gently onto the upper shoulders. Make sure that pressure is not put on the head and neck.

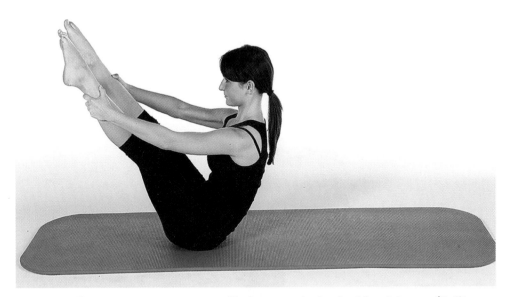

Inhale and roll up to starting position and balance on the back of the sit bones. (Rolling forward of the sit bones will cause you to lose the elongated C curve.)

Perform 6 times.

Note
Only practice this exercise on a surface that gives ample cushioning for the spine. A mat that is at least ¾″ thick is recommended.

The Cork-Screw (Modification: Torso on Mat)

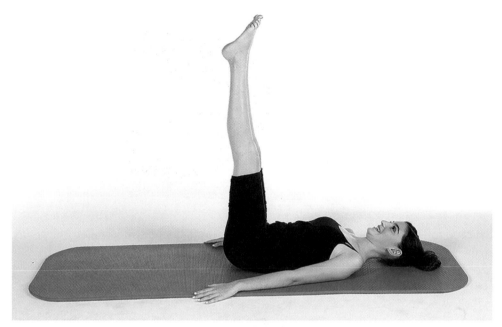

Lie supine with head resting on the mat. Press arms down on the mat alongside the body. Extend legs toward ceiling keeping hips on mat. Inhale and exhale.

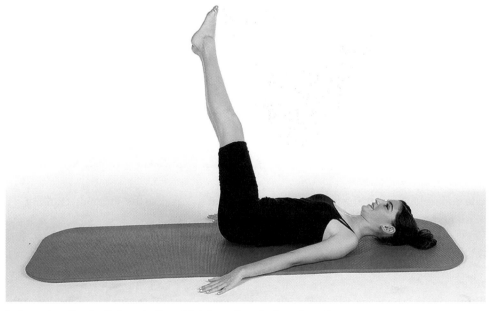

Inhale, extending both legs to the right, keeping the legs together.

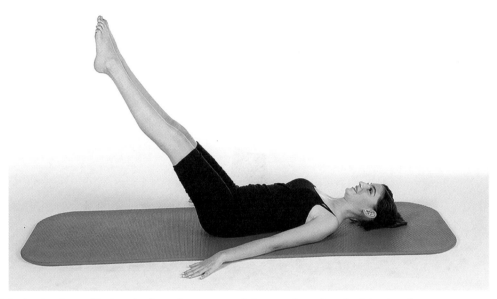

Exhale slowly and bring the legs down toward the mat keeping the hips level.

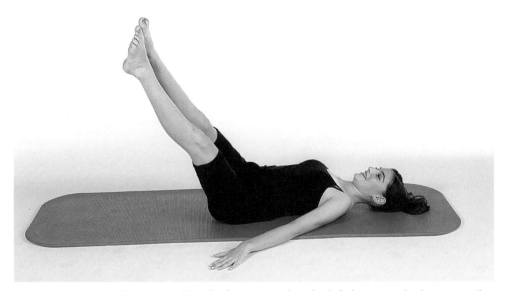

Continue the exhale while extending the legs around to the left, bringing the legs up to the start position.

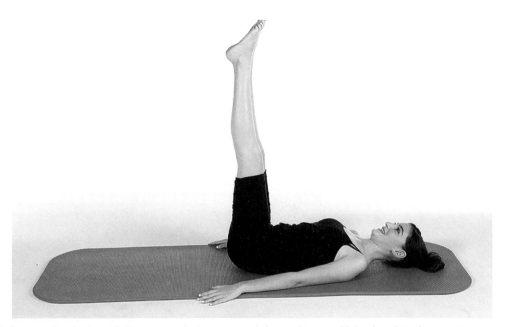

Inhale and exhale with legs extended up toward the ceiling and hips level in the starting position.

Begin this cycle again going to the left side first.
Perform 3 cycles in each direction, alternating right and left.

Modification
Try the exercise keeping legs in table top position.

The Saw

Keep the hips square to the front and both sit bones on the mat throughout the exercise.

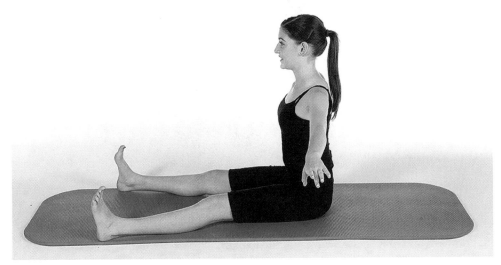

Sit on the mat with the spine long as if up against a wall. Extend legs in front of the body, with flexed feet apart, slightly wider than hip width. Extend arms out to the sides and slightly in front of the shoulders.

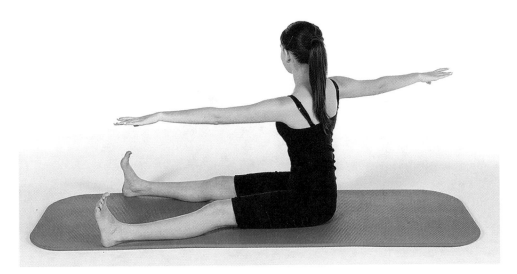

Inhale and rotate the upper torso to the right.

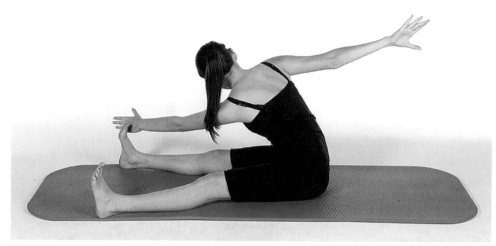

Exhale and round the spine forward over the right leg. Reach the left arm toward the right foot, and cross left hand over right ankle, alongside the outside of the right foot. Reach the right arm back and diagonally away from the left arm. Look toward the back arm.

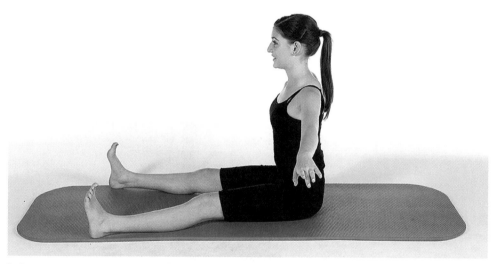

Inhale to untwist and sit upright. Exhale and stay.

Repeat entire exercise to the left.

Perform 3 times on each side.

Modification
If the student has tight hamstrings, they can sit on a rolled up mat or block for better spinal alignment.

Note
The focus of this exercise is rotation and flexion of the spine, to improve spinal mobility. Avoid overstretching the hamstrings or forcing students to reach to or past their foot.

Imagery: Imagine wringing the air out of the lungs like wringing water out of a wet towel.

The Neck Pull

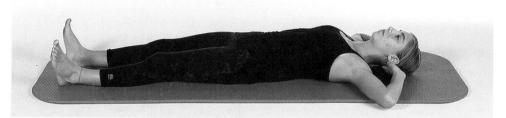

Lie supine with fingers interlocked behind the head. Aim elbows slightly forward, to avoid rib flaring. (As a variation, try opening the elbows as widely as possible, without letting the ribs flare.) Legs are straight on the mat in parallel, either hip width distance apart or together, with feet flexed.

Imagery: Imagine the feet pressing into a wall.

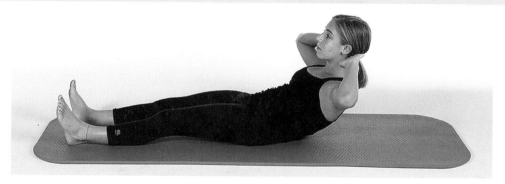

Inhale to lengthen the back of the neck and upper back. Exhale and roll the head and the back of the rib cage off the floor into a forward curl. Lengthen and traction the back of the neck with the hands.

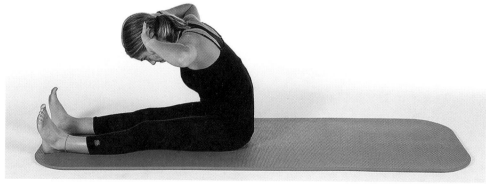

Continue to exhale and to roll forward until in The Spine Stretch position.

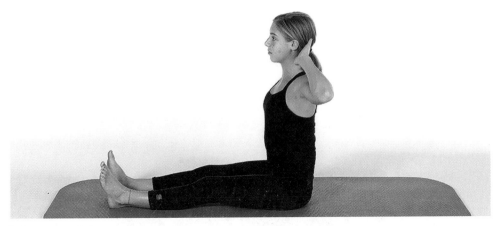

Inhale to unroll the trunk into a tall, seated position.

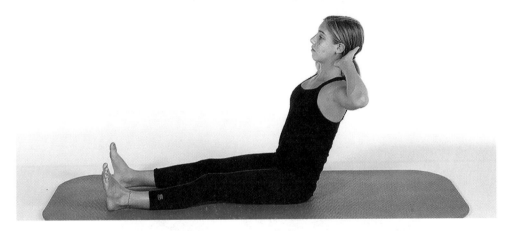

Continue inhalation and hinge back.

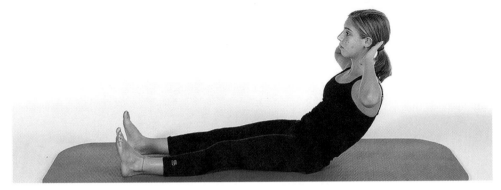

Exhale and begin to roll down, from the sacrum, through the torso, returning to start position.

Perform 3 to 5 times.

Modification
Reach the arms forward, or cross the hands on the elbows in "genie" position.

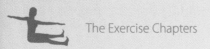

The Side Kick

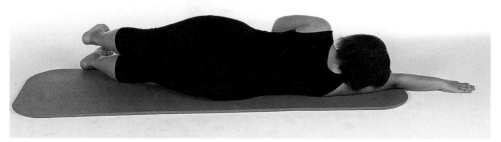

Lie on your side. Align the head, upper back, and pelvis in a straight line. Stack the top shoulder and hip directly on top of the bottom shoulder and hip. Place the legs forward of the hips about 2 feet.

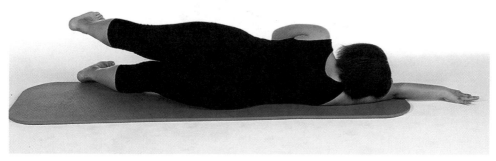

Slightly turn out the bottom leg, and lift the top leg parallel to the mat. Rest the head on the bottom arm, (arm straight or bent). Rest the top arm along the body or press the hand flat on to the floor in front of the body for balance. Slightly lift the right side of the waist off the mat.

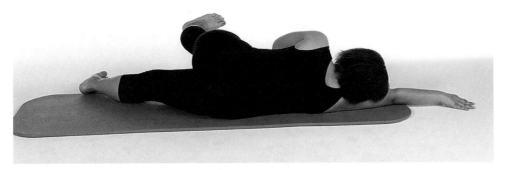

Inhale, and swing the top leg forward.

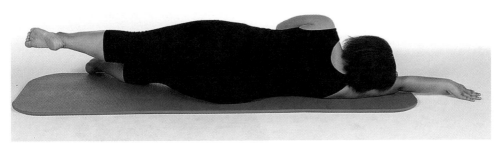

Exhale, swing the leg back. Keep the torso stable and still while the top leg moves forward and back.

Perform 6 to 10 swings front and back. Focus on length and stability of the torso and the moving leg throughout exercise.

Note
As an alternative experience, try exhaling on the forward swing, and inhaling on the backward swing.

Imagery: Move the leg like a pendulum. Move the leg as if moving through the arc of **a** rainbow.

Criss Cross

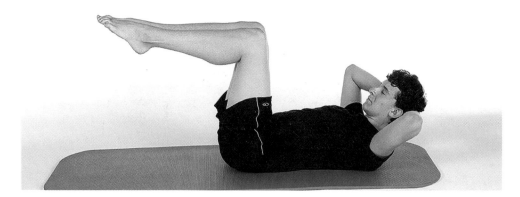

Lie supine. Bend legs into table top position, with the feet and knees together. Place hands behind the base of the head, fingers interlaced. Inhale, and lengthen back of the neck and upper back, and roll the head and the back of the rib cage off the floor into a forward curl.

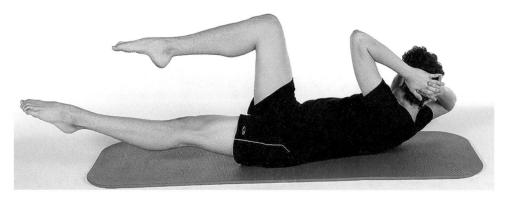

Exhale and twist the upper body to the right. Aim the left shoulder toward the right knee and straighten the left leg.

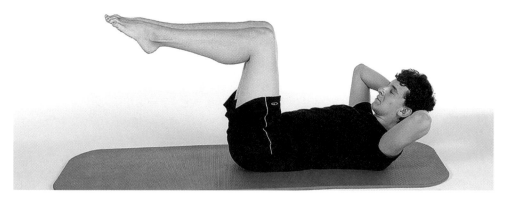

Inhale and return to start position.

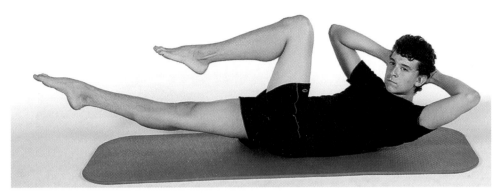

Exhale and twist the upper body to the left. Aim the right shoulder toward the left knee and straighten the right leg.

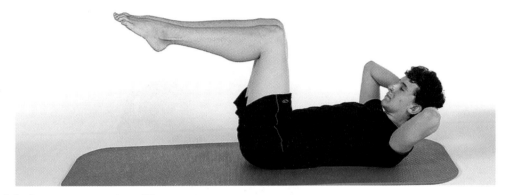

Inhale, return to start position.

Perform 5 times each side.

Note

As an alternative experience, try alternating the breathing pattern.

Progression

Alternate side to side without stopping in the table top position.

The Teaser

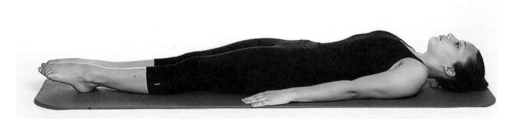

Lie supine. Lengthen arms and legs on mat, palms facing down, legs parallel and together. Feet pointed.

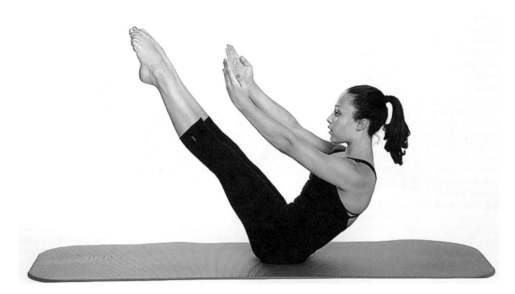

Inhale, lengthen the back of the neck and roll up into The Teaser "v" position, balance behind the sit bones near the bottom of the sacrum. Reach the arms toward the toes. Exhale slowly while holding the position. Inhale at the top of position.

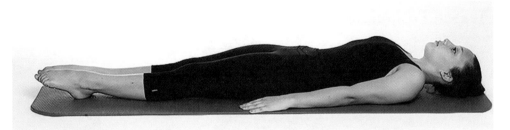

Then exhale and begin to roll back through the pelvis and torso, lowering the legs until lying flat on the mat.

Perform 3 times.

Note
Keep the spine in a long flexion curve while in The Teaser position.
Avoid spine extension or an anterior pelvic tilt.

Imagery: Visualize the body as a hammock suspended from two palm trees.

Modification
As a modification you may do a "Single Leg Teaser", keeping one leg bent at the knee and planted securely on the floor as shown in the previous chapter.

The Teaser (Progression: Moving the Torso)

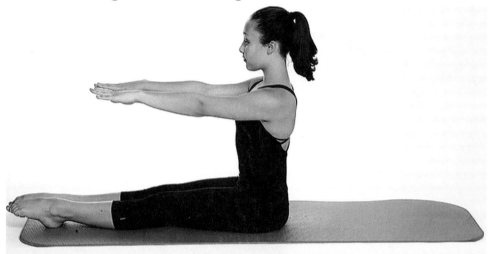

Sit in a long sit position with the legs together and arms reaching forward. Inhale slowly and grow taller.

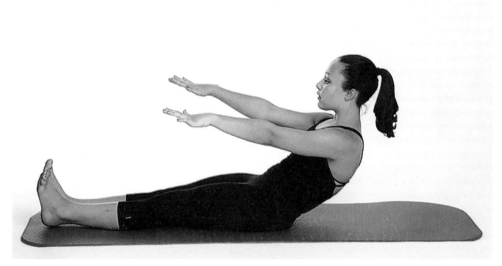

Exhale slowly and roll back through the pelvis and spine.

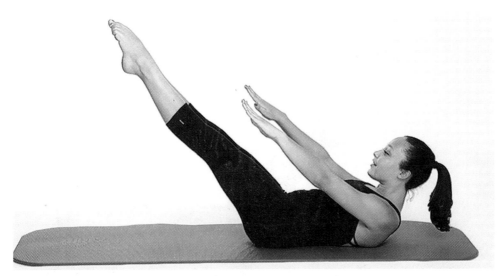

During the roll-back, lift the legs to 45 degrees.

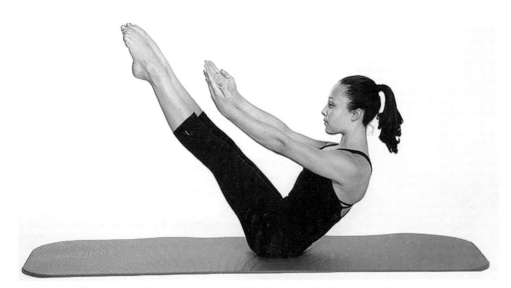

Inhale and roll up to The Teaser position while keeping the legs at 45 degrees.

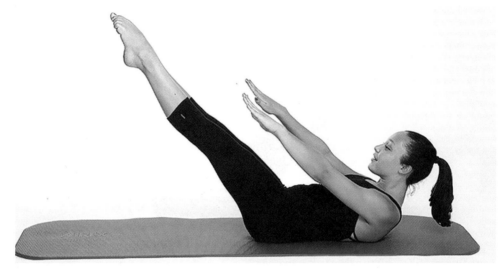

Exhale and roll back, keeping the legs at 45 degrees.

Perform 3 to 5 times.

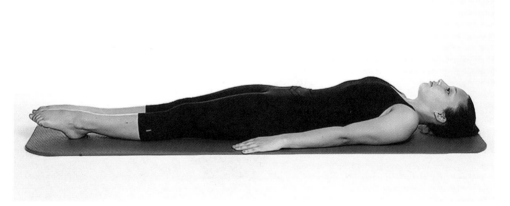

Then roll down to supine position to finish and rest.

Note
Arm height and leg height remains consistent while rolling up and down.

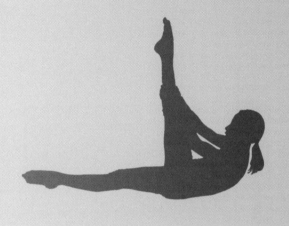

Section Three
Curriculum

Chapter 10
Curriculum for Schools

Curriculum Presentation

For those Pilates teachers who wish to initiate and implement a Pilates program within a school, it is essential to be prepared to make a successful presentation to school administrators who will approve or reject the proposal. The proposal should take the form of a written 'curriculum'. In formal education, a curriculum outlines the planned interaction of students with course content, materials and resources, and the processes for evaluating whether or not the educational objectives have been met.

> *The curriculum presentation should be designed so that a busy teacher or administrator can read it quickly, absorb the key points being made, and make an informed decision about the proposal. As such, it should be clear and compelling.*

The curriculum should be no longer than a few pages, with the information presented in a tidy, succinct manner, using bullet points or tables to focus the reader's eye on the most important information. Ideally, it should be tailored to the individual school or district where the course is to be taught. Therefore, if possible, it is advisable for the Pilates teacher to have a conversation with the local principal, school head, or classroom teachers who may provide insight into the school's priorities, resources and facilities. For example, it might be possible to include Pilates classes within a school's existing Physical Education or Health curriculum. Alternatively, a school may only want Pilates within their program for part of the year, or as an after school program. Having this information will aid in the preparation of a successful curriculum presentation. Know your audience and their expectations before presenting your proposal.

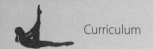

Curriculum Content

The school administrator making the decision to approve or reject the curriculum proposal will need to review basic facts about the Pilates program being proposed. While there is no set format for written curriculums, the Pilates teacher should consider including some or all of the content below to structure the proposal for a specific school.

- Introduction/Overview
- Target age level
- Timing: Length of course (e.g. 12 weeks, or academic year) and lessons (e.g. 50 minutes)
- Materials required (mats and/or other materials)
- Rationale
- Aims, goals and objectives
- National Standards addressed for Physical Education
- Course content (overview of course of lessons)
- Sample lesson plans
- Funding required (If funds are available, they may come from school budgets or a Parent Teacher Association (PTA). The proposal should elicit a "yes" with regard to funding.)
- Assessment methods

Sample Curriculums

Two sample curriculums follow below, as examples of how the presentation may be done. It is important to bear in mind that the curriculum presentation can be tailored as the Pilates teacher sees fit, in order to best meet the needs or address the priorities of the target school.

Note

While mats that are a minimum of ¾" thick are essential for participation in a Pilates class, the Pilates teacher should bear in mind that for some schools, the need for equipment or props may be a barrier to acceptance of the proposal, due to cost. The Pilates teacher should consider whether props are integral to the lesson plan, and whether or not they can provide them if the school cannot. It is important to remember that it is possible to create excellent lesson plans for young people based solely on the Pilates exercise repertoire and imagery.

Proposal – Sample A

PILATES COURSE CURRICULUM

INTRODUCTION

I propose to teach a Pilates program at (school name) for 5th graders (approximate ages 10-11). The course will last for 12 weeks, and will consist of one 50-minute lesson per week. Each child will require a mat that is at least ¾" thick. Failure to use mats of the appropriate thickness may cause injury.

RATIONALE

The reason to implement this program is to teach children strategies to enhance or maintain their overall health and to improve their quality of life. Pilates exercises improve children's strength, flexibility, balance, stability, coordination, concentration, posture, bone density, joint health, and breath capacity. Pilates breathing techniques serve to relax the body and to calm and focus the mind, and are extremely helpful for students' performance both in the school environment and in the rest of life. The curriculum is specially designed to be developmentally appropriate for children, and to foster body awareness and self-confidence.

AIMS

The aim of this curriculum is to educate children about their bodies, to provide them with a positive, non-competitive movement experience, and to establish healthy exercise habits. The curriculum aims to produce physically literate individuals, as per the National Standards below.

NATIONAL STANDARDS FOR K-12 PHYSICAL EDUCATION

- **Standard 1** - The physically literate individual demonstrates competency in a variety of motor skills and movement patterns.
- **Standard 2** - The physically literate individual applies knowledge of concepts, principles, strategies and tactics related to movement and performance.
- **Standard 3** - The physically literate individual demonstrates the knowledge and skills to achieve and maintain a health-enhancing level of physical activity and fitness.

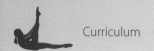

- **Standard 4** - The physically literate individual exhibits responsible personal and social behavior that respects self and others.
- **Standard 5** - The physically literate individual recognizes the value of physical activity for health, enjoyment, challenge, self-expression and social interaction.

(http://www.aahperd.org/naspe/standards/nationalStandards/)

OBJECTIVES

- Students will experience how Pilates breathing can relax the body, and calm and focus the mind.
- Students will learn movement sequences that establish efficient movement patterns in their bodies.
- Students will perform exercises that heighten their vestibular and proprioceptive senses.
- Students will practice exercises to achieve greater strength, flexibility, agility, balance, and stability.
- Students will practice exercises to achieve better posture and coordination.
- Students will practice exercises to maintain joint health, bone density, and to increase breath capacity.
- Students will be able to identify specific parts of the human muscular and skeletal system.
- Students will be able to identify key movement principles of the Pilates Method of body conditioning.

COURSE CONTENT

This curriculum explores the principles of the Pilates Method by focusing on the *movement principles* of:

- Whole Body Movement
- Breathing
- Balanced Muscle Development
- Concentration
- Control
- Centering
- Precision
- Rhythm

The body is organized to move by *centering*. *Balanced muscle development* allows efficient movement and proper joint mechanics. Constant mental *concentration* is required to fully develop the body. *Precision*, meaning exact, defined, specific, intentional movement, is necessary for correct form. Only a few repetitions of each exercise are appropriate so that each repetition can be performed with the greatest *control*, using only the necessary muscles and effort necessary for each movement. *Breathing* promotes natural movement and *rhythm,* and stimulates muscles to greater activity. Performance of the Pilates exercises is distinguished by always using the *whole body*. (The PMA Pilates Certification Exam Study Guide, 2014).

FUNDING REQUIRED

$X/session for Pilates teacher x 12 weeks = $Y

ASSESSMENT METHODS

- Execution of tasks assessed via rubric (see top of next page)
- Journal writing
- Exit Slips. (Each student is given an Exit Slip printout with a question about the day's lesson. Students are asked to write their responses and hand them to the teacher before leaving class.)

Sample rubric

Area	Excellent 1	Very good 2	Good 3	Needs work 4	Score
Execution of the Pilates mat exercises	Engaged and concentrated when executing the Pilates mat exercises. Improves very rapidly.	Engaged when executing the Pilates mat exercises. Improves rapidly.	Executes the Pilates mat exercises. Improves.	Does not try to execute the Pilates mat exercises. Does not improve.	
Body	Significant increase in strength, flexibility, balance, stability, coordination and posture. Very attuned sense of body awareness.	Good increase in strength, flexibility, balance, stability, coordination and posture. Good sense of body awareness.	Increase in strength, flexibility, balance, stability, coordination and posture. Has some sense of body awareness.	Does not increase in strength, flexibility, balance, stability, coordination, or posture. Low sense of body awareness.	

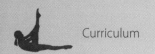

CONCLUSION

According to the National Association for Sports and Physical Education (NASPE): "The goal of physical education is to develop physically literate individuals who have the knowledge, skills and confidence to enjoy a lifetime of healthful physical activity." (http://www.aahperd.org/naspe/standards/nationalStandards/) A Pilates curriculum will address and exceed the national standards for K-12 physical education, while teaching students to embody the Pilates Method of body conditioning, which will support their participation in study, work and play.

Proposal – Sample B

PILATES COURSE CURRICULUM

INTRODUCTION

This curriculum explores the principles of the Pilates Method by focusing on the movement principles of whole body movement, breathing, balanced muscle development, concentration, control, centering, precision, and rhythm.

Pilates improves strength, flexibility, balance, stability, coordination, posture, bone density, and breath capacity. The goal of Pilates instruction is to improve one's overall quality of life.

According to the National Association for Sports and Physical Education (NASPE): "The goal of physical education is to develop physically literate individuals who have the knowledge, skills and confidence to enjoy a lifetime of healthful physical activity." (http://www.aahperd.org/naspe/standards/nationalStandards/) A Pilates curriculum will address and exceed the national standards for K-12 physical education, while teaching students to embody the Pilates Method of body conditioning, which will support their participation in study, work and play.

COURSE OBJECTIVES

- Participate in an exercise program to increase strength, balance, and flexibility.
- Become familiar with the Pilates Method, its benefits and movement principles.
- Understand and experience the benefits of practicing Pilates breathing.
- Increase body-mind integration.

COURSE DESCRIPTION

In this course, students will be introduced to the 34 mat exercises outlined in Pilates' book, *Return to Life*. Students will also explore the fundamental Pilates movement principles that underlie proper performance of all Pilates exercises. The course is designed to assist participants in establishing strength and stability, improved coordination, balance, posture and flexibility, and a heightened sense of body-mind integration. Emphasis will be placed on reaching an intermediate level of execution of the exercises, with precise alignment, proper breathing, and efficient sequencing of movement.

This comprehensive course explores musculoskeletal anatomy and basic kinesiology principles—emphasizing the trunk, hip, shoulder girdle, arm, and neck—as they relate to the teaching and practice of Pilates. This course is presented in a lecture and

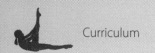

practice format. Throughout the course, students gain hands-on experience via regular palpation of their own muscles, bones, and ligaments. Additional topics such as core stability and the anatomical basis of common tension patterns are also addressed.

CLASS FREQUENCY AND AGE GROUP

The course will consist of 2 classes per week, offered over 9 weeks, making a total of 18 classes. The course is designed for high school students in the 11th or 12th grades (approximate ages 15 – 18).

COURSE RESOURCES
Printed handouts
Book: *Return to Life*, by Joseph Pilates

EQUIPMENT REQUIRED
Mats, fitness circles, weighted balls, flex bands and stability balls.

COURSE OVERVIEW
Week 1

Discussion: What is the Pilates Method? What are its benefits? What are the basic movement principles delineated in *Return to Life*? Introduce pre-Pilates exercises.

Week 2

Discuss breathing and pelvic placement during Pilates exercise. Discuss the benefits of regular Pilates practice. Begin Pilates practice.

Week 3

Continue Pilates practice. Discuss alignment and flexibility. Delineate key muscle groups, their actions, and how they can work together to create stability and balance.

Week 4

Further explore Pilates movemement principles while continuing to practice Pilates exercises. How can the movement principles be identified within each exercise?

Week 5 & Week 6

Continue Pilates practice and review of movement principles along with anatomy review as related to exercise repertoire.

Week 7

Raise the level of exercise execution to intermediate level, include transitions, and focus on awareness of movement principles while performing exercises. Emphasize the benefits of Pilates breath work.

Week 8 & Week 9

Practice Pilates exercises at intermediate level, and review the physical skills attained throughout the course.

FUNDING REQUIRED

$500 – for fitness circles, weighted balls, flex bands and stability balls

ASSESSMENT

- Demonstration of correct practice
- Journaling
- Projects

SAMPLE LESSON OUTLINE

- Lecture: What is Pilates? What are its fundamental movement principles?
- Discuss major muscle groups and the concept of core strength and control.
- Demonstrate exercises and begin teaching movement
    - Pre-Pilates; Warm-Up
    - Exercises
    - Cool-Down
- Assign reading, writing, exercise practice, or other homework

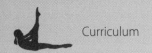

Sample Parent Letter

Parents serve as primary educators, and any opportunity that allows for a partnership between the school and the parents enhances the learning experience for students. Some schools will wish to communicate directly with parents about a new program such as Pilates, and the sample letter below is one way to ensure support and understanding. Providing a letter such as this to the school administrator (in case they need it) makes their job easier and may help in having the proposal approved.

Date

SAMPLE

Dear Parents,

At (*insert name of school*), we believe it is important to educate the whole child. Developing healthy habits and positive attitudes in relation to exercise improves the overall quality of life of the child. Beginning on (*insert date*), (*insert name of school*) will start teaching a Pilates class to students (*insert frequency*). The program is intended to provide students with a positive, non-competitive movement experience, focusing on improving strength, balance and flexibility. Pilates exercises improve stability, coordination, and posture, as well as joint health and breathing capacity.

(Suggestion: Introduce the Pilates teacher and their background. Be brief.)

Should you have any questions or concerns, or if you do not want your child to participate in the Pilates program, we ask that you contact (*name of contact*) at the following (*email address or telephone number*) by (*date*) so that we can discuss your decision further.

Thank you for your support of our efforts to create a healthy tomorrow.

Sincerely,

(Name of School Principal)   (Name of Pilates Teacher / Classroom Teacher)
Principal   Pilates Teacher / Classroom Teacher

Sample Lesson Plans

Sample lesson plans for early childhood, middle childhood, and adolescence are included below to help stimulate the Pilates teacher's imagination in designing a complete program based on age-appropriate activities. The Pilates teacher will need to plan these lessons in advance of each class, and be able to show the plans to school adminstrators, although detailed plans for each lesson are not required for a curriculum presentation.

Early Childhood – Sample lesson plan

The Snake Lesson

Ideal ages: 5–7

Learning objectives

After exploring different ways that a snake can move, by the end of the lesson students will have identified descriptive vocabulary words that they can relate to a variety of snake-like movement sequences.

Assessment

I will know that the learning has been achieved by the students' ability to use the descriptive words and demonstrate the associated actions that we have identified in class.

Duration of Class

30-40 minutes.

Materials

Wooden toy snake, mats, balls, scarves, large paper, markers

Preparation/Special Management/Job Helpers:

- Mats will be pre-set in a circle formation in the room
- Balls and scarves will be ready for use
- Job helpers will help to supply balls and scarves when needed

Entrance strategy

I will have the students stand in a single file line, with their hands on the shoulders of the person in front of them. In the single line, the students will slowly snake through the classroom exploring the space and the various floor pathways that they can design. The students will end in a circle on the mats.

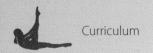

Motivation

I will start by introducing the students to my new pet, Sylvester, who is an articulated toy snake made of wood.

Lesson introduction/focus exercise

I will have the students pass Sylvester around the circle. Each student explores how Sylvester moves.

Guided question

"Can you say some words that describe how Sylvester the snake moves?"

Lesson introduction

I will write down action words that describe how snakes can move on large pieces of paper, and will then have the students use their bodies to interpret the words.

Warm-up

Snake Breath: Have the students inhale, and then have them extend the exhalation as long as they can, making a hissing sound like a snake.

Exploration

- Standing position, rolling down and up – Articulate the spine down and up
- Use Snake Breath
- The Rollup, using a ball – coiling and uncoiling in and out
- Rolling Back (Rolling like a Ball)– Keeping the body in a tight snake coil
- Swan Dive Preparation, with a ball – Extend the spine up like a cobra (Lie prone, with hands extended over head on a ball, roll the ball toward the body and extend the spine up. Then roll the ball away from the body and allow the spine to roll down.)
- Spine Stretch Forward – Articulate the spine like a snake articulates its spine when it slithers.

Development

Snake Charmer Activity

I will pull a scarf out of my sleeve and let them know that I'm going to charm them like a snake, having them mirror the scarf's movements.

Creating/sharing

Once the students have the idea of mirroring the action of the scarf, I will then break them into pairs, giving each pair a scarf. One student takes the role of the charmer, while the other takes the role of the snake. After a period of time they switch roles. Each student receives equal time with both roles.

Conclusion/reflection
Cooling-down Wiggle exercise
I will guide students through their anatomical landmarks and have them gently wiggle these various landmarks to release tension from their bodies.

Exit strategy
Students will re-form a single file line, with their hands on the shoulders of the person in front of them. In a single line, the students will slowly snake their way out of the classroom space.

Middle Childhood – Sample lesson plan

The Three-Movement Circus
Ideal ages: 8–9

Learning objective
After exploring how movement occurs in three dimensions (in the sagittal, coronal and transverse planes), by the end of the lesson students will be able to identify the three dimensions and give examples of movement in each dimension.

Assessment
I will know that the learning is achieved by the students' demonstration of a correct use of sagittal, coronal, and transverse dimensions dimensions in different movement phrases.

Duration of class
45–55 minutes

Materials
Mats, yellow, green and red tape, balls, circus music

Preparation/Special Management/Job Helpers
- Mats will be pre-set in a circle formation in the room
- All props will be pre-set
- Yellow, green and red circles will be pre-taped to the floor
- There will be special job helpers to guide the class into different stations as well as job helpers to collect the mats and balls.

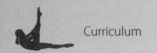

Entrance strategy

"Statues". The teacher counts the students off one-by-one to enter the classroom on the count of 4. "1, 2, 3, 4, Go! 1, 2, 3, 4, Go! 1, 2, 3, 4, Go!" The student runs in, finds an empty space on the floor and strikes and holds any pose they'd like, like a marble statue.

Warm-up, selected exercises

- The Hundred, modified versions and progressions
- The Roll Up
- The One Leg Circle (with knee bent)
- Rolling Back
- The One Leg Stretch
- The Double Leg Stretch
- Criss-Cross, modified versions
- The Spine Stretch

Motivation

I will start by rolling and bouncing balls on and across the floor.

Guided question

"How and in which ways are these balls moving, and in which directions?"

Lesson introduction/focus exercise

Have the students move via forward and backward pathways. Have the students notice how they are moving in space, as well as which body parts are moving to accomplish the given task. Do the same with moving up and down, as well as across and side-to-side.

Exploration

The students explore moving front and back, up and down, across and side-to-side, using quick or sustained and strong or light movement qualities.

Development

Have the students swallow an imaginary ball, and tell them to picture the imaginary ball moving through their bodies, making them perform movements in the three different dimensions.

Creating/sharing

Divide the class into pairs. Each person must develop a short phrase that moves in one of the three dimensions, and then teach their partner the phrase. There will be three circles taped on the floor in different colors, representing each dimension. Yellow will represent sagittal, green will represent coronal and red will represent transverse. The students must guess which dimension of movement the sequence their partner created represents, and memorize the movement routine. Students will perform their routines in pairs in the appropriate circle, so that no one performs alone. The class will assess if they have picked the correct circle. Circus music will be played as they perform.

Conclusion/reflection

The students will cool down by returning to their partners and mirroring each other using any movements in any dimension. Students will take turns being the leader and follower.

Exit strategy

I will call the students one by one and have them run, jump and give me a "high five" as they exit. The last two students will be called together, so that no one is last.

Adolescents – Sample lesson plan

Moving from the Center Out

Ideal ages: 14–18

Learning objective

To draw a parallel between the way the planets of the solar system rotate around the sun and how the peripheral body parts extend from and rely on the trunk of the body. Students will deconstruct Pilates exercises, exploring movement initiations.

Assessment

I will know that the learning objectives are met by the students' teaching and demonstration of the deconstructed Pilates exercise sequences.

Duration of Class

45-55 minutes

Materials

Styrofoam planets, string, thumb tacks,

Preparation/Special Management/Job Helpers

I will have the classroom set up with models of the sun and planets of our solar system hanging from the ceiling.

Motivation

I will have the students walk around the room observing the different parts of the solar system and how it is organized.

Guided questions

"What is the center of our solar system?" "If we think of the human body as a metaphor for the solar system, which part of the body would the sun be?"

Lesson introduction/focus exercise

I will have the students review the fundamental movement principles of Pilates, with an emphasis on the principal of "centering". I will then have the students explore moving from distal to core, and from core to distal (from the center out).

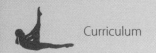

Warm-up, selected exercises

The Hundred	The Cork-Screw (modified)
The Roll Up	The Saw
The One Leg Circle	The One Leg Kick
Rolling Back	The Double Leg Kick
The One Leg Stretch	The Neck Pull
The Double Leg Stretch	The Side Kick
Criss-Cross	The Teaser (modified)
The Spine Stretch	Swimming
Rocker with Open Legs	The Seal

Exploration

I will take three exercises from the warm-up and deconstruct some of the movement components, highlighting what the movement might look or feel like when it is initiated from core to distal and when it is initiated from distal to core.

Development

I will break the students into pairs, working with the same three exercises. I will have them explore, with their own bodies, how it feels to execute the exercises initiating movement from core to distal and how it feels to execute the exercises initiating movement from distal to core.

Creating/sharing

I will divide the classroom into four groups and give them a teaching exercise. I will have each group choose one exercise from the warm-up that has not been deconstructed and have them deconstruct the exercise's sequence of movements with regard to: what initiates, what follows, and how it can be done initiating the movements from core to distal. They will share their findings with the rest of the class.

Conclusion/reflection

I will have them finish by brainstorming to think of other objects that are the vital center of a structure or unit (like the sun in the solar system); for example, a keystone of a bridge, or a trunk of a tree.

Assessment will consist of

- Exit slips
- Journal writing
- Peer evaluation in various activities
- Execution of a task

Conclusion

By following the guidelines in this chapter regarding the curriculum presentation process, the Pilates teacher should be able to create an effective proposal for their target school that stands a strong chance of being accepted by school administrators. Undertaking informal research into the target school's priorities, resources and facilities will help the Pilates teacher make strategic decisions about how to prioritize information within the proposal that will be relevant and meaningful to the school decision-makers. We hope that the two sample curriculums in this chapter will provide a useful roadmap for designing curriculum presentations tailored to the target school. It is important to remember that there is no standard format for such curriculums. Therefore, it is best to approach curriculum writing with a clean slate for each school, bearing in mind the unique conditions of the target school and the need to communicate the basic information that administrators will require to inform and support their decisions.

We hope that, over time, finding Pilates programs in schools for all age groups will become the norm. The benefits of the Pilates Method can be made available to children and adolescents during the school day if Pilates teachers and school administrators work together to adapt Pilates programs for the large variety of school environments that we find in the world today.

In closing, let us remember this message from Joseph Pilates in his book, *Return to Life*:

"With body, mind, and spirit functioning perfectly as a coordinated whole, what else could reasonably be expected other than an active, alert, disciplined person? (Pilates, 1945)."

Fostering the well-being of young people through the practice of the Pilates Method will encourage the healthy functioning and joyful living of tomorrow's adults.

Appendix 1

Pilates in the Schools – Healthy Habits for Life

Launched in 2003, the PMA's school-based health and wellness program, Pilates in the Schools - Healthy Habits for Life, was designed to create an opportunity for young people to experience the mental, physical, and emotional fitness benefits inherent in the Pilates Method.

The program's primary goal was to bring Pilates to children and adolescents, by providing affordable and accessible Pilates education to schools. The program was intended to include all young people regardless of their environment or background, based on the belief that a program of this kind can potentially create a global shift in the health and wellness of our youth. A series of program pilots was initiated between October of 2004 and November of 2008, and produced results for the participants in the areas of core strength, hamstring flexibility, and balance. The pilots targeted 5th and 6th graders, (approximately ages 9 to 13), based on the idea that this age range represented the "magic window" of opportunity for creating healthy habits for life. The Pilates in the Schools approach was rooted in the idea that whole body wellness must embrace the whole person/whole child perspective.

Pilates instructors from a variety of cities throughout the US followed PMA protocols for setting up a program pilot and conducted pre- and post-pilot measurements in order to collect data documenting the outcomes of the pilots.

The pilots were structured as a series of sessions of 45 to 50 minutes in length, taking place over a period of 10 weeks. Students learned specific physical skills while developing awareness of their bodies, incorporating the elements of focused awareness, concentration, coordination, healthy breathing, and mindful and controlled movement. The pilots were designed by selecting a specific set of Pilates-based exercises that were deemed appropriate and safe for children at the 5th and 6th grade level. The exercises targeted key areas of physical and cognitive development, and were correlated with the California Department of Education Standards in addition to universally accepted health and wellness principles validated by contemporary medical and science-based research.

The intention of the simple but specific pilot design was to create measurable positive outcomes through a curriculum that would foster mental fitness, emotional and physical well-being, and social competence.

The pilots' objectives were realized through a series of group sessions with the following pedagogical focus:

- **Body Positioning and Awareness Skills** (focused awareness, attention, and concentration), to shift the student's focus from external stimuli to internal awareness of where the body is in space.
- **Healthful Breathing** techniques, to promote slowing down, reflecting and becoming present.
- **Coordinated Breathing,** to coordinate breathing patterns with movements and identify how the breath can make movements easier or harder.
- **Core Strengthening** exercises, to strengthen the core muscles; to support healthy growth and development of the trunk and extremities as well as to develop awareness of how using the core muscles can assist with a variety of other sport and non-sport activities.
- **Flexibility,** to identify the presence or absence of flexibility in key muscle groups which contribute to a healthy postural balance within the body.
- **Concentration and Coordination,** to assist the development of focused movement and concentration through choreographed sequences of movements with changing tempos.
- **Relaxation**, to promote balance and calm.
- **Group Discussion,** to allow students an opportunity for inquiry and comment.

Pilot Outcomes

The program pilots were designed to create measurable outcomes, as well as to foster mental fitness, emotional and physical well-being, and social competence.

The areas of measurement for physical outcomes were:
1. Flexibility
2. Strength
3. Balance

Simple tests were devised, and data were collected before and after the Pilates pilots. The results are set out in the graphs below. The data show significant improvements in all test results over the (average) 10 week pilot.

Forward bend

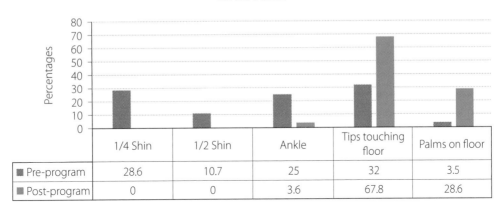

	1/4 Shin	1/2 Shin	Ankle	Tips touching floor	Palms on floor
■ Pre-program	28.6	10.7	25	32	3.5
■ Post-program	0	0	3.6	67.8	28.6

Push-up position hold

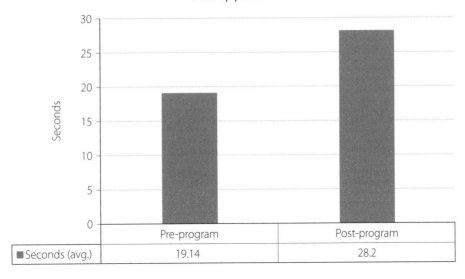

	Pre-program	Post-program
■ Seconds (avg.)	19.14	28.2

Single leg stand

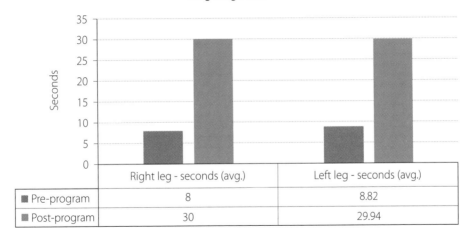

	Right leg - seconds (avg.)	Left leg - seconds (avg.)
■ Pre-program	8	8.82
■ Post-program	30	29.94

Pilates Tools for Teachers

Pilates Tools for Teachers (PTT) was a one-day training course designed to teach schoolteachers how to use Pilates in the classroom to facilitate a variety of different learning objectives. This course was directed not at Pilates teachers, but at schoolteachers with no previous Pilates experience.

PTT was created in response to requests from classroom teachers who had identified improved behaviors in their students who had participated in the pilots, and were interested in using Pilates exercises in the classroom. The purpose of PTT was to provide a methodology whereby Pilates skills developed in the pilots could be practiced and reinforced in the classroom as life tools for focus, concentration, learning readiness, stress management, health, and self-management.

PTT trained schoolteachers to lead 5 to 10 minute Pilates-based exercise sequences, designed to integrate mindful physical activity, self-awareness, relaxation and creativity. It enabled schoolteachers to provide regular exercise and mind–body integration activities which could be done in the classroom setting.

Appendix 2

Working with Young People with Special Needs

The World Health Organization defines "disabilities" as an umbrella term encompassing impairments, activity limitations, and participation restrictions. Young people with disabilities or special needs can benefit from the positive effects of a Pilates-based movement program.

Physical fitness is especially important for young people with special needs as they move towards puberty and adulthood. Consistent exercise helps equip them with tools for navigating the physical and emotional challenges that their developing mind and body may experience. Each student should have a unique age-related fitness program as outlined in this manual, in addition to their own therapeutic goals. By working as part of a student's team and maintaining regular communication with their physical and/or occupational therapists, the Pilates teacher can assist in guiding appropriate programming for their specific needs.

A thorough medical screening and clearance from the student's doctor is essential before they participate in any kind of specialized exercise program. It is important that all members of the student's healthcare team be informed and in agreement with the student's participation in a Pilates-based movement program.

The decision to work with special populations must be clearly based in the teacher's scope of practice and experience as a movement educator. Self-education through the Internet or books is not a substitute for continuing education, practical experience, and observation of licensed healthcare practitioners, recreational therapists, and credentialed teachers.

As we have seen in this manual, working with children and adolescents must not be approached in the same way as working with adults. Children who have unique challenges and needs due to neurological, musculoskeletal, emotional, or cognitive function deficits require even greater consideration when designing a Pilates-based movement program.

Exercise has positive effects on the brain (van Praag, 2009). In general terms:

- Exercise modulates the body's physiological response to stress.
- Focused breathing initiates the relaxation response and improves receptivity of the nervous system.
- Pilates exercises activate and integrate all of the body's systems to encourage an energized, alert state.
- Exercise places the brain into a state of homeostasis and balances the body's chemistry, organ and electrical systems, which can help reduce stress in children and improve their overall well-being.
- Exercise has a similar effect on the body to antidepressant medications, without drugs.

The two most significant benefits of Pilates for children with unique challenges are:

1. Pilates promotes whole-brain function for optimal learning.
2. Focused breathing and physical activity increases circulation, which boosts the flow of oxygen and glucose to the brain and body.

The Pilates principles discussed in the following paragraphs have benefits for young people of all levels of function.

Pilates Movement Principles and their Benefits for Young People with Special Needs

Focused breathing and concentration during movement, as practiced in Pilates, can allow students to slow down and to identify the effects of breath on movement. As the difficulty of an exercise increases, breath coordination becomes increasingly important. Young people learn to coordinate breathing patterns with movement by executing Pilates exercises with precision and control. The increased level of concentration that this requires assists in conditioning the nervous system and encouraging its overall coordination for optimal movement.

Learning about control through Pilates exercise can be extremely liberating for many children and adolescents with disabilities. Being perceived as "different" is potentially distressing for a young person. By learning to control specific aspects of the exercises, Pilates can bring about a sense of strength and empowerment.

Practicing Pilates exercises with precise body positioning and movement helps to develop focused awareness, attention, and concentration. These skills are valuable for shifting focus from external stimuli to internal awareness of the body in space.

Pilates exercises condition the muscles of the torso, which supports good posture, healthy growth, and development of the trunk and extremities. Learning Pilates can build awareness of how the deep muscles of the trunk can assist with a variety of functional activities which many children with disabilities find challenging.

By suggesting self-assessment questions, the teacher can assist the student in making discoveries about their own body mechanics. Identifying flexibility and strength (or the lack thereof) in the key muscle groups that enable balanced posture can be highly encouraging to students with physical challenges, in a way that pointing out individual differences between students is not.

Choreographed sequences of movements with changing tempos assists in the development of focused movement and concentration, and positively impacts neurological functioning for young people with special needs.

In addition to the positive effects of Pilates movement principles, young people with physical or developmental challenges will find Pilates beneficial through the cultivation of relaxation and the use of the breath. A young person's use of relaxation skills in Pilates to promote balance and calm affects how they respond to all of life. An awareness of the difference between breath to facilitate work and breath to facilitate relaxation increases their knowledge of the different uses of breath.

Effects of the Pilates Method on Common Physical, Cognitive and Sensory Challenges

Hypotonicity (a state of decreased or low muscle tone)

Although all of Pilates can be deemed beneficial for young people with special needs, the benefits of breathing work and the stimulation of BDNF, (a protein secreted in the brain), are particularly noteworthy for children and adolescents with low muscle tone.

Increased blood flow stimulated by breathing in the practice of Pilates movements assists with the delivery of oxygen and glucose, which are essential for heightened alertness and mental focus.

When children undertake physical activity, a protein known as BDNF (brain-derived neurotrophic factor) is secreted in the brain. BDNF acts on certain neurons of the central and peripheral nervous systems, in areas vital to learning, memory, and higher thinking. The flow of BDNF decreases after 20 minutes of sitting, and is triggered again by movement. Children with moderate to severe hypotonia (decreased muscle tone) are often fitted with specialized seating systems and sit for very extended periods of time, thereby inhibiting the production of BDNF.

Exercises that are particularly helpful for young people with low muscle tone:
- The Bridge
- The Hundred
- The Double Kick
- The One Leg Kick

Hypertonicity, (a state of increased or excessive muscle tone)

Diane Damiano (Dodd et al., 2002) has studied and written about the importance of strength training for children with spasticity, a form of hypertonicity. Appropriate weight-bearing through the long bones helps to maintain bone density and joint structure, which may be compromised as a result of spasticity.

Exercise and strengthening are important for a young person with hypertonic movement dysfunction, to prevent overuse of the strong muscles, atrophy and wasting of weaker muscles, and obesity. (O'Shea, 2009).

Exercises that are particularly helpful:

- The Roll Up
- Rolling Back (Rolling Like a Ball)
- The One Leg Stretch
- The Double Leg Stretch

Attentional Dysfunction

Achieving homeostatic balance (the state of internal equilibrium) for this group of young people is very important for their overall physical and emotional health. Exercise such as Pilates helps shift the body-brain into a homeostatic state – balancing brain chemistry, hormones, and the functioning of all the body's systems. In addition, recent research has demonstrated that exercise can provide many benefits for young people, such as decreased stress, anxiety, and depression. Exercise has also been shown to improve symptoms of ADHD (attention-deficit/hyperactivity disorder) such as negative affect, poor impulse control, and compulsive behavior. Finally, research has correlated exercise with improved executive functioning, working memory, and reduced stress levels for relatives and care-givers of young people with ADHD (Archer and Kostrzewa, 2012).

As described previously, Pilates promotes improved function in key areas of the brain such as the basal ganglia, cerebellum, and corpus callosum, by building brain cells and neural connections (Lin, 2012). These areas have been identified in research as regions that, when stimulated, have a direct effect on decreasing some of the symptoms associated with ADHD. The Pilates principles of concentration, focus and movement precision during exercise promote the integration and harmonizing of the mind and the body. This integration of the mind and body during movement encourages task efficiency and mental focus for young people with ADHD. Directed or cued physical activity prior to concentration tasks has been shown to stimulate the frontal lobe of the brain, enhancing memory, creativity and academic achievement (Caterino and Polak, 1999).

Sensory Integration Challenges

Many young people with sensory integration challenges have a difficult time processing and integrating input from the environment. Physical exercise such as Pilates can work to increase their self-awareness. The use of directed imagery or mental images combined with Pilates exercises increases mind and body awareness, which can improve overall function for these young people. This carries over into self-care and management skills.

The regular practice of Pilates enhances the integration of the vestibular (balance), cerebellar (balance and muscle coordination), and reticular activating (attention) systems. This integration is critical to improving attention and coordination, both physically and cognitively. Young people with sensory integration challenges tend to be highly kinesthetic in their orientation to the environment. Exercise has been shown to help students who are kinesthetic learners (Hannaford, 1995), and therefore young people with sensory integration issues stand to benefit from Pilates. For all of the reasons discussed above, the teaching of Pilates to young people with special needs is a logical application of this amazing work within a specific context. Implementing successful Pilates programs for this special population highlights its benefits for people of all levels of function.

References

Archer, T., Kostrzewa, R. M., 2012. Physical exercise alleviates ADHD symptoms: regional deficits and development trajectory. *Neurotoxicity Research*, 21(2):195–209

Caterino, M. C., Polak, E. D., 1999. Effects of two types of activity on the performance of second-, third-, and fourth-grade students on a test of concentration. *Perceptual and Motor Skills*, 89(1):245–248

Dodd K. J. et al., 2002. A systematic review of the effectiveness of strength-training programs for people with cerebral palsy. *Archives of Physical Medicine and Rehabilitation*, 83(8):1157–1164

Hannaford, C., 1995. *Smart moves: Why learning is not all in your head*. Salt Lake City, Great River Books

Lin, T.W et al., 2012. Different types of exercise induce differential effects on neuronal adaptations and memory performance. *Neurobiology of Learning and Memory*, 97(1):140-7

O'Shea, R., 2009. *Pediatrics for the physical therapist assistant*. Edinburgh, W.B. Saunders

Van Praag, H., 2009. Exercise and the brain: something to chew on. *Trends in Neuroscience*, 32(5):283–290

Appendix 3

Pilates Philosophy and Principles

Joseph Pilates' philosophy, as stated in his 1945 book *Return To Life through Contrology*, is a vision of health and well-being that gives context to his exercises. The Guiding Principles are essential for teachers to understand in order to carry forth Pilates' intended purpose.

The Three Guiding Pilates Principles

- Whole Body Health
- Whole Body Commitment
- Breath

Whole Body Health

"Physical fitness is the attainment and maintenance of a uniformly developed body with a sound mind fully capable of naturally, easily, and satisfactorily performing our many and varied tasks with spontaneous zest and pleasure (Pilates, 1945)."

"Whole Body Health" refers to the development of the body, the mind and the spirit in complete coordination with each other. Pilates wrote that "Whole Body Health" could be achieved through exercise, proper diet, good hygiene and sleeping habits, plenty of sunshine and fresh air, and a balance in life of work, recreation and relaxation.

Whole Body Commitment

"To achieve the highest accomplishments within the scope of our capabilities in all walks of life, we must constantly strive to acquire strong, healthy bodies and develop our minds to the limit of our ability (Pilates, 1945)."

"Faithfully perform your Contrology exercises only four times a week for just three months...you will find your body development approaching the ideal, accompanied by renewed mental vigor and spiritual enhancement (Pilates, 1945)."

"Whole Body Commitment" is mental and physical discipline, a work ethic, an attitude toward one's self and a lifestyle that is necessary to achieve "Whole Body Health".

Breath

The breath is an integral part of overall body functioning, increasing volume capacity, oxygenation and other physiological changes. Full consistent inhalation and exhalation helps the circulatory system nourish all the tissues with oxygen-rich blood while carrying away impurities and metabolic waste. Pilates referred to this cleansing mechanism as the "internal shower" which resulted in mental and physical invigoration and rejuvenation.

The Pilates Movement Principles

The Movement Principles are elements that are present in the successful performance of all the Pilates exercises:

- Whole Body Movement
- Breathing
- Balanced Muscle Development
- Concentration
- Control
- Centering
- Precision
- Rhythm

The body is organized to move by *centering*. *Balanced muscle development* allows efficient movement and proper joint mechanics. Constant mental *concentration* is required to fully develop the body. *Precision*, meaning exact, defined, specific, intentional movement, is necessary for correct form. Only a few repetitions of each exercise are appropriate so that each repetition can be performed with the greatest *control*, using only the necessary muscles and effort necessary for each movement. *Breathing* promotes natural movement and *rhythm* and stimulates muscles to greater activity. Performance of the Pilates exercises is distinguished by always using the *whole body*.

Goals and Benefits

> *"One of the major results of Contrology is gaining the mastery of the mind over the complete control of your body (Pilates, 1945)."*

The Guiding Principles and Movement Principles facilitate long-term goal achievement. The benefits are both measurable and perceived:

- Coordination
- Strength
- Mobility
- Efficient movement
- Flowing movement
- Proper posture
- Mental and spiritual rejuvenation
- Self-awareness
- Self-confidence
- Restoration of natural animal movement
- Integration of mind, body and spirit
- Sense of well-being
- Enhanced quality of life

Reference

Pilates JH, Miller WR., 2005. *Return To Life Through Contrology*, Miami: Pilates Method Alliance, Inc. Reprinted with permission from *The PMA Pilates Certification Exam Study Guide*, 2014. Miami: Pilates Method Alliance, Inc. Available from the PMA: www.pilatesmethodalliance.org

Appendix 4

PMA Code of Ethics

PMA Members and PMA Certified Pilates Teachers must abide by these guidelines:

1. Do no harm.

2. Teach within the "Scope of Practice."

3. Maintain professional boundaries:
    a. No inappropriate physical contact
    b. No financial exploitation
    c. No sexual exploitation

4. Maintain client confidentiality.

5. Direct clients to seek medical attention when necessary.

6. Do not discriminate.

7. Do not knowingly solicit other Pilates professionals' clients.

8. Treat clients and colleagues with respect, truth, fairness and integrity.

9. Comply with all applicable business, employment and intellectual property laws.

10. Maintain professional appearance and conduct.

11. Do not misrepresent skills, training, professional credentials, identity or services.

12. Continue education to enhance skills and knowledge, in order to provide highest quality services to your clients.

Appendix 5

PMA Scope of Practice

PMA members and PMA Certified Pilates Teachers must work within the scope of practice of a Pilates teacher as outlined below:

The following is within the scope of practice of a Pilates teacher

1. Design Pilates exercise programs according to an individual's needs.
2. Recognize conditions that would preclude a client from safely participating in Pilates exercise program.
3. Coach, provide general information, and direct clients to seek medical attention as necessary.
4. Receive exercise guidelines for clearance from medical practitioners when appropriate, to ensure client's safety.
5. Document client's progress and cooperate with referring medical practitioners.
6. Promote exercise to improve overall health.
7. Request permission to touch clients and observe practice laws within the jurisdiction.
8. Use appropriate touch to facilitate movement, position the client, and to prevent injury or damage.

The following is beyond the scope of practice of a Pilates teacher

1. "Prescribing" an exercise program.
2. "Diagnosing" a client with any medical, mental, or physical condition.
3. Continuing to train a client who has a condition beyond your knowledge without appropriate medical clearance.
4. "Prescribing" diets or recommending supplements.
5. Claiming to "treat" or "rehabilitate" injury or disease.
6. Monitoring (measuring with instrumentation) the progress of clients referred by therapists or medical practitioners.
7. Offering counseling.
8. Claiming to be competent to offer professional education beyond the limits of your credentials.
9. Applying inappropriate touch.
10. Continuing to train a client that exhibits any of the following unusual symptoms: chest pain, prolonged dizziness, rapid heart rate, shortness of breath, significant decrease in coordination, loss of consciousness, faintness, nausea, blurred vision, prolonged or increasing pain.

Index